THE

CUPPING

BOOK

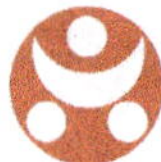

Jun Zi Publishing

info@thecuppingbook.com
http://thecuppingbook.com
907 S Lakewood Ave
Baltimore, MD 21224

ISBN: 979-8-218-26709-4 (paperback)
ISBN: 979-8-218-28510-4 (ebook)

Library of Congress Control Number: 2023917949

Printed in Baltimore, Maryland

Ordering Information:
Special discounts are available on quantity purchases by corporations, associations, and others. For details, contact info@thecuppingbook.com, http://thecuppingbook.com, http://charmcityintegrative.com
443-869-6584
907 S Lakewood Ave
Baltimore, MD 21224

Names: Ingegno, Tom, 1977- .

Title: The cupping book : unlocking the secrets of ancient healing / Dr. Tom Ingegno, DACM, LAC.

Description: Baltimore, MD : Jun Zi Publishing, 2024. | Includes color photos and diagrams. | Includes bibliographical references. | Summary: Presents the history of cupping and the actual practice at home for various health conditions. Includes step-by-step instructions with photos.

Identifiers: LCCN 2023917949 | ISBN 9798218267094 (pbk.) | ISBN 9798218285104 (ebook)

Subjects: LCSH: Cupping. | Cupping — Handbooks, manuals, etc. | Alternative medicine. | Medicine, Chinese. | BISAC: MEDICAL / Alternative & Complementary Medicine. | HEALTH & FITNESS / Alternative Therapies. | BODY, MIND & SPIRIT / Healing / General.

Classification: LCC RM184.I54 2024 | DDC 615.89 I--dc23

LC record available at https://lccn.loc.gov/2023917949

THE CUPPING BOOK

UNLOCKING THE SECRETS OF ANCIENT HEALING

DR. TOM INGEGNO, DACM, LAC

You Got Sick—Now What?
Seven Secrets from Oriental Medicine
to Eliminate the Cold and Flu

Disclaimer:

This book details the author's experiences with and opinions about cupping therapy. The author is not your healthcare provider. The author and publisher provide this book and its contents on an "as is" basis and make no representations or warranties concerning this book or its contents. The author and publisher disclaim all such representations and warranties, including, for example, warranties of merchantability and healthcare for a particular purpose. In addition, the author and publisher do not represent or warrant that the information accessible via this book is accurate, complete, or current.

The U.S. Food and Drug Administration has not evaluated the statements about products and services. They are not intended to diagnose, treat, cure, or prevent any condition or disease. Please consult your physician or healthcare specialist regarding the suggestions and recommendations in this book.

Except as expressly stated in this book, neither the author nor publisher, any authors, contributors, or other representatives will be liable for damages arising from or in connection with the use of this book.

This is a comprehensive limitation of liability that applies to all damages of any kind, including (without limitation) compensatory, direct, indirect, or consequential damages; loss of data, income, or profit; loss of property or property damage; and claims of third parties.

You understand that this book is not intended as a substitute for consultation with a licensed healthcare practitioner, such as your physician. Therefore, before you begin any healthcare program or change your lifestyle, you will consult your physician or another licensed healthcare practitioner to ensure that you are in good health and that the examples in this book will not harm you.

This book provides content related to physical and/or mental health issues. As such, using this book implies your acceptance of this disclaimer.

DEDICATIONS

To my wife, Maura-Leigh, and my daughters, Chloe and Mabel:

You have blessed my life with the most powerful of all medicines, *love*. I cannot put into words how much you mean to me. I love you beyond life itself.

To my late mentor and friend, Peter Yates:

I still hear your words daily. I am striving to follow my own path and honor all the practitioners that came before me. Your impact on so many students who have become friends and family reaches globally, and even though you have passed across the veil, your work and mission will be carried on forever. I owe you a debt I can never repay.

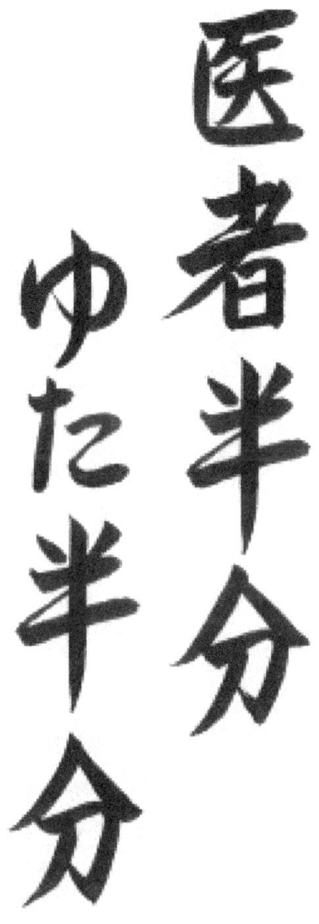

ISHA HANBUN YUTA HANBUN

"When seeking advice seek both a doctor and a shaman."

Direct translation: "Half Doctor, Half Shaman"

Calligraphy by Eri Takase, StockKanji.com

FOREWORD

"Life, liberty, and the pursuit of happiness," or so it says in the Declaration of Independence. I love the Declaration of Independence. It is a tad wordy, but otherwise, it is obviously a pivotal document for our country. I like this phrase the best, though, as it perfectly summarizes some of our most valued ideals.

While there is an infinite array of ways one could interpret this, I genuinely believe that the bedrock of happiness is our health. In a modern age where hunting is no longer a requirement and our basic survival needs are primarily met with ease, we do not see boundless happiness in the world. In fact, things are trending in quite the opposite direction. As it seems, health is the ultimate privilege, which was relegated to the wealthy elite not so long ago, the educated elite after that. Presently, it resides primarily in the hands of tech giants and well-connected "influencers."

As the founding fathers said, these are unalienable rights. And yet we find ourselves no longer chasing life, liberty, or the pursuit of happiness, but rather clinging to life through means that are alien to us as a species. Many are glued to computer screens by necessity due to work, others for the allure of entertainment, and some are simply losing themselves in the virtual world, all at the expense of meaningful engagement in the physical world and, all too often, at the expense of their own personal health (physical and mental).

This concept is not recent; humanity has pursued these ideals in various forms for millennia. Intrinsically, we are built to drive toward these goals. And why not? These are fundamental not only to our minds, bodies, and souls, but, even if we had no name or description for them, they would be fundamental to sustaining life itself.

Despite living in an age where we have a near-infinite capacity to acquire data, we routinely fail to do so in the realm of our own health and wellness. The connection between us and our physical world continues to erode. This has spawned a slew of modern illnesses and maladies. Despite being alive in a time with unprecedented medical advancements, we are sicker than we have ever been. After stalling out for centuries, the maximum lifespan finally nearly doubled in the 20th century.[1] It subsequently saw a significant two-year decline in 2021 and 2022, the biggest decline in the last 100 years.[2]

On *Irreverent Health*, Tom and I regularly discuss optimization of one's health, in particular, the importance of taking personal control over your own health. We don't do this because it is easy, but rather because it is the only reliable way in this modern

---

1   Steven Johnson, "How Humanity Gave Itself an Extra Life," *New York Times Magazine, April 27, 2021,* https://www.nytimes.com/2021/04/27/magazine/global-life-span.html.
2   "Life Expectancy in the U.S. Dropped for the Second Year in a Row in 2021," Centers for Disease Control and Prevention, August 31, 2022, https://www.cdc.gov/nchs/pressroom/nchs_press_releases/2022/20220831.htm.

age to know for sure you are doing all you can to optimize your own health. Also, we do it because we love it. I mean, we really, really love it. It is that shared love of endlessly examining various modes of health augmentation that draws me to Tom's work again and again.

Outside of the show, I have worked with Tom on various self-health projects such as cryotherapy, salt therapy, exercise with oxygen therapy (EWOT), infrared sauna, and red light therapy. His overall knowledge of these "alternative" modes of healing is encyclopedic and would impress even the staunchest stoic. That said, working with him on cupping was, to say the least, transformative. In near-immediate fashion, Tom was able to identify, explain, and treat an issue that had haunted me for years. The result was so profound and so immediate that I joked it was magic. Well, I said it was a joke, anyway. On the inside, it was nothing short of magic to me.

This is why Tom's work holds such significance for me. It perfectly shines a light on the two things Tom brings to the table in spades: a herculean knowledge of acupuncture, cupping, and Chinese medicine as a whole and a capacity to distill said knowledge into language anyone can comprehend. Tom has found a way to bind an otherwise foreign and esoteric modality into something that is as easy to understand as ordering a Big Mac—something modern denizens of, well, Earth, can understand and assimilate into their lives with nearly zero barriers.

For anyone looking to learn more about cupping today—like, right now—this book is for you. If you have tried other ways to self-heal and struggled, you would not be the first. This book should be the de facto field guide for cupping as it provides easy-to-understand wisdom that is immediately actionable.

As we begin to explore new ways to improve our health, these pockets of wisdom will be increasingly useful. I applaud Tom for taking the time to distill this down into such a densely valuable work that even Luddites like myself can wrap their heads around it. I wish everyone who uses this book amazing success and continued health.

Matt Hampton

Cohost on the *Irreverent Health* podcast

TABLE OF CONTENTS

PREFACE

As long as humans have been humans, we have searched for ways to feel better. While discoveries in medicine happen at a daily pace today, humans haven't changed much since we started living in agricultural societies. While we must continue our efforts to advance medicine as far as possible, it's also imperative that we don't throw the proverbial "baby out with the bathwater" when looking at long-standing traditional practices.

I began my studies in East Asian medicine in 1998. Quickly, I learned that these traditional practices not only held up to modern scientific scrutiny, but in many cases surpassed the benefits of state-of-the-art standards of Western medical care in side-by-side scientific studies. Attempts to disprove these practices through the gold standards of double-blind, placebo-controlled studies simply served to confirm the wisdom and complexity of a medical system that dates back well over 4,000 years.

If there is modern validity for East Asian practices, what clinical pearls might have been abandoned from other long-standing practices? Will traditions be lost to time, or can we resurrect those beneficial procedures that provide important benefits to this day? These questions have stuck with me since my first theory class on my career path to becoming an acupuncturist. It is my intention to shine light on some of these practices that are both traditional and evidence based.

Cupping is the most widely practiced traditional therapy across cultures and ages. It has been a familiar healing technique in homes across the globe and has been passed on from generation to generation without dwindling into the common historical commentary of, "look at how foolish our ancestors were, thinking we could heal ourselves with an obscure practice like that." In my tenure as an East Asian medicine practitioner, I have seen cupping therapy re-emerge as a common practice that has practitioners of many different licenses trying to claim it as their own. In truth, although licensed healthcare practitioners receive training in cupping, its safety, effectiveness, and ease of application make it one of the most accessible homecare practices available.

With that said, I am inviting you, dear reader, to join me on an exploration of our shared history and to learn how to perform cupping at home with modern style cups. I hope to continue my education in these traditional practices and share what is safe and effective with the world. I would like to thank you in advance for choosing this book and to wish you success with this powerful healing method.

INTRODUCTION

"If there was something excellent to be used as a remedy,
then it is hijama [cupping]."

—BOOK 31, HADITH 41 FROM SUNAN IBN MAJAH 3476

A BIT ABOUT ME

I have been an acupuncturist and integrative medicine practitioner for more than two decades and have dedicated myself to assisting others in maintaining and expanding their health. While patients are on my table, I use various techniques and therapies to help stimulate their body to restore natural function and correct injuries and illnesses.

In treating patients over the years, I've noticed one factor that always contributes to achieving positive results is their willingness to practice some form of care at home. Keeping to a regular treatment plan and showing up to appointments is good, but during the time between treatments a patient can either aid their progress or hinder it. Some of the things that can help their condition include exercise, stretching, medicinal herbs, supplements, prescription medications, meditation, and *qigong* (a system of breathing and movement exercises that helps to circulate energy through the body). Of course, this list is not exhaustive. A range of traditional therapies—many of which have passed through generations—can also be performed safely at home to aid in healing oneself.

Perhaps the oldest and most widely spread of those traditional therapies is cupping. I didn't realize quite how wide its geographical use was until I taught at the Pacific College of Oriental Medicine in New York City where I had many international students. Regardless of a student's heritage, when the conversation turned to cupping, they would say, "Grandma used to do that."

I encourage anyone reading this book to follow the long history of home practitioners and continue the traditional practice that our common ancestors started nearly 4,000 years ago. Today, we can use modern cupping tools to make it easier and safer to help ourselves and our loved ones feel better.

WHAT IS CUPPING THERAPY?

If you've been to a gym, watched any of the last three summer Olympics, or followed any health-minded celebrity on social media, no doubt you have seen perfectly circular temporary "bruises" on a person's body. The name of this effective practice—cupping—suggests the use of some type of cup, and practitioners often say how amazing it feels. Cupping therapy claims benefits from pain relief to stimulating "detox."

WHAT EXACTLY IS CUPPING?

The most straightforward explanation is that cupping is a therapeutic technique that uses a vacuum created inside a cup to help improve circulation and increase space between the skin, fascia (connective tissue), and muscles. The "space" created by the cups allows inflammation to emerge from deeper tissue. It can be recirculated to the body's core to be processed while pulling fresh blood into the area to allow healing and relax muscles. In addition, the new blood has oxygen and nutrients that bathe the surrounding area, relieving pain and repairing tissue. The "bruises," known as ecchymosis, occur as the vacuum pulls the skin and ruptures the tiny capillaries at the surface.

We could do a deep dive into the role of fascia, modern-day research, and how inflammatory markers such as cytokines cause pain and disease. However, this book is meant to be practical and hands-on and will allow you to "hit the ground running" with cupping and allow for self-treatment and the treatment of friends and family. Plus, unless you're a researcher or clinician, discussion of the inflammation process can be pretty dull.

In its most traditional form, which varies throughout the world, cupping uses an open flame to consume the oxygen in the cup and create the vacuum. Many modern cupping devices don't require an open flame and are safer and generally easier to apply outside of a clinical setting. With the wide variety of cupping sets and styles available, you have many options for performing cupping on yourself and friends effectively.

My mentor often repeated the classical Chinese adage, "When drinking water, remember the source." With that in mind, this book will provide you with all the basics you need to know about cupping. You will learn:

- A little of its history and how it is used today

- How and why it is performed and how it can improve different aspects of your life

- How to apply cupping to help relieve aches and pains for yourself and others

- How each style of cupping device works and how to shop for the device that's best for you

A BRIEF HISTORY OF CUPPING THERAPY

"When drinking water, remember the source."

—CHINESE PROVERB

As a doctor of acupuncture and Chinese medicine, I'd love to think that acupuncture is the oldest healing modality, at least as a formalized system. Yet, in recorded history, cupping has more than 1,000 years on acupuncture.

Cupping's origin story is a little murky. It isn't entirely clear which country or civilization first developed the technique, but the most likely suspects are ancient Persia, Greece, or Egypt. The *Eber's Papyrus,* dating from Egypt, circa 1550 BC, one of the oldest medical texts on record, discusses cupping. Persian physicians discussed cupping, or *hijama,* heavily in *The Cannon of Medicine (Al-Qanun fi al-Tibb,* 1025 BC). The prophet Mohammed mentioned cupping often in the Koran, and many Muslims still perform cupping during Sunnah days for health and religious observation today. The Greeks discussed it frequently, and the "father of modern medicine," Hippocrates, compiled significant writings on cupping therapy.

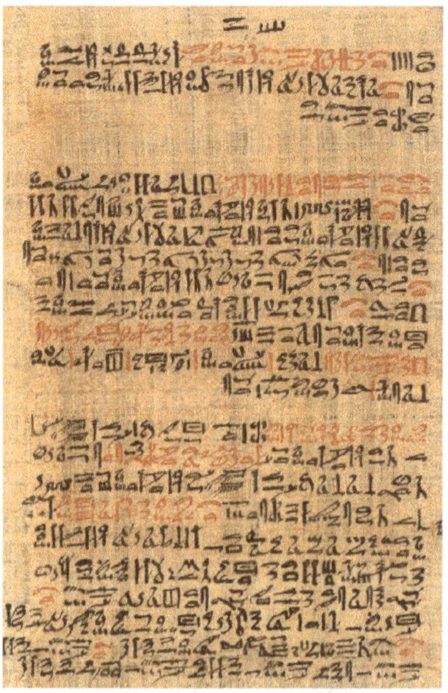

A Page from the Eber's Papyrus

One of these civilizations may have been responsible for cupping becoming a near-global presence in the ancient world. Although how the technique spread is unclear, it's probable that it reached Asia, Africa, Europe, and Russia via silk trade routes. Interestingly, South America also developed a cupping system called *Ventosa*, which has an equally long history of therapeutic use. It's fascinating to consider whether South America developed cupping separately or if the ancient world wasn't as isolated as we think.

In ancient China, doctors of traditional Chinese medicine knew cupping well and considered it a home therapy for patients to apply before seeking professional help. However, it wasn't until roughly AD 300 that a famous Chinese physician, Ge Hong, discussed cupping in his text, *Prescriptions for Emergencies*, as a

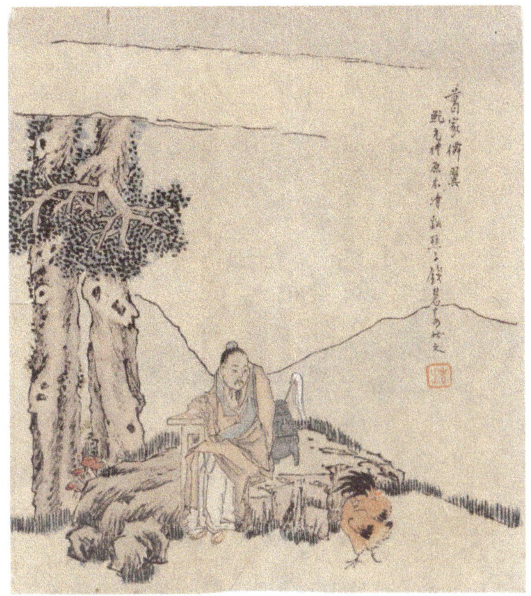

Ge Hong (Ko Hung, 283—343 CE)

treatment that physicians should employ in their clinics. It was almost as if he was saying, "Hey guys, get off your high horses. This stuff works."

In ancient societies, the first cups were made of animal horn, sections of bamboo, or clay, and fire created the suction necessary to adhere cups to the skin. As glass production became more common, people used household cups and cups explicitly designed for therapy. These usually had a thick lip to provide more comfort when applied. Modern-day cups are made of a variety of materials. There are glass cups, but the best home-use sets might be those made of plastic or silicone, which can use a pump, bulb, screw-top, or press to create the vacuum.

Other evolutions in cupping methodology include multiple therapies such as heat, electric stimulation, magnets, vibration, and

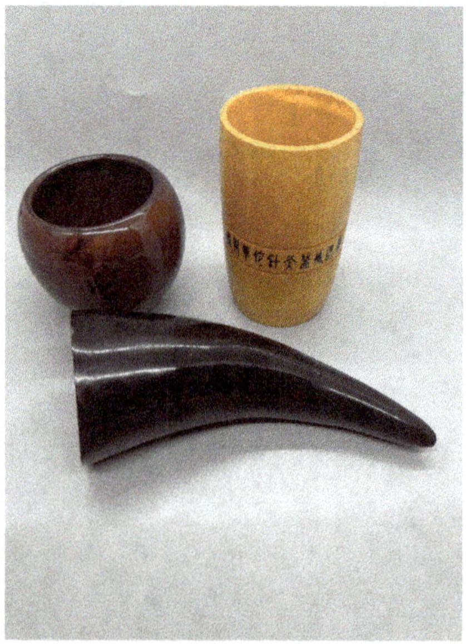

Traditional Cupping Tools

red-light therapy. As most of my current practice focuses on combining treatments in an organized way, a process I refer to as "stacking," I'm excited to see these multiple-intervention-based home devices. (Worry not! I already have another book in the works on the concept of stacking!)

Cupping has had several moments in the limelight in recent years in the United States. In 2006, Gwyneth Paltrow wore a backless dress to a red-carpet movie premiere. Yes, the dress was gorgeous, but the buzz around her photos was all about the perfectly circular bruises running from her shoulders to her hips on full display. It only took one look at the pictures in news outlets for me to add the words "cupping therapy" to the other services I list on my clinic's sign. I quickly learned of nail salons and spas in Los Angeles charging more than $200 for a quick cupping session. If only Grandma knew, she could have made a fortune!

Paltrow may have gotten the ball rolling—at least she got parts of the Western world interested in what many other countries were already doing. Olympian swimmer Michael Phelps mainstreamed cupping in 2016 when he dove into the water to collect gold medals while rocking the signature marks all over his built-perfectly-for-swimming body. The buzz was so big within a day after his first event that local TV news reporters were in my Baltimore office reporting about how Phelps—our hometown hero—loves cupping. (The clip is on my clinic's YouTube channel; remember to like and subscribe. ☺)

While that event etched cupping in Americans' minds, anyone who already knew about cupping would have noticed signs of it in the previous 2012 Olympics. Of course, Michael Phelps was front and center then too, giving interviews to journalists from the pool while plenty of Asian swimmers with the telltale circular marks on their skin lined up behind the journalists asking Phelps the same canned questions regarding his abilities and how it feels to represent America.

Even before Phelps brought this therapy front and center in the U.S., it wasn't entirely out of the public eye as immigrants from around the globe brought many of their traditional healing practices with them to this country. With the prevalence of cupping in traditional medicine, there's no way cupping couldn't have found a home in the U.S. In fact, it had enjoyed a little time in the limelight long before Phelps was out of swimmy diapers. The 1964 classic film *Zorba the Greek* demonstrated cupping, and Nonna in *The Godfather II* (1974) performed cupping on the infant, Fredo, for a respiratory condition that had made him weak.

All this attention to cupping in the last decades drove manufacturers to develop new cupping devices and reach a broader range of customers. In 2014, I prototyped cups that made a heart and a diamond-shaped mark on a patient's back.

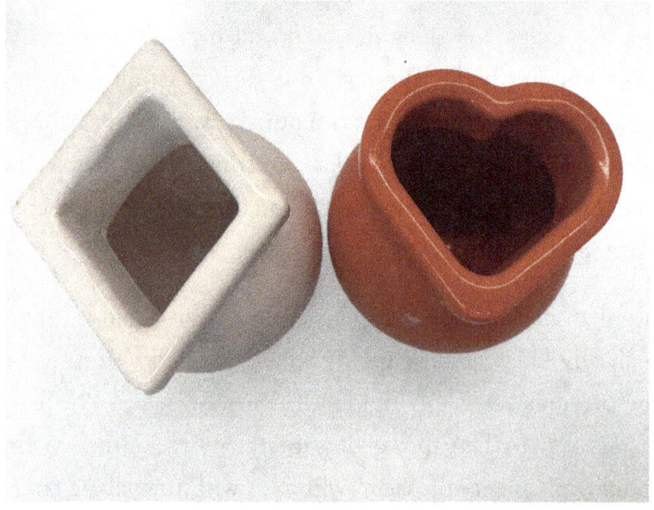

Novelty Shaped Cups prototyped by the Author

Then I got a phone call from a colleague who attended a conference that mentioned another acupuncturist was working on the same idea. I guess she saw the writing on the wall as well. Sadly, someone beat me to the market. However, I knew others would copy this new cup style once one person made it. Within six months, more companies made heart shapes and stars. No doubt, there will be more shapes and sizes soon. While I may have missed my window to jump on a product idea, all these companies seizing this opportunity prove that cupping has become mainstream. It only took about 4,000 years.

WHY LEARN CUPPING THERAPY?

Traditional healing interventions often work best at the first signs of a problem. Professional treatments can provide better relief, but being able to apply cups whenever you need them is a great benefit. Since cupping is fast and overwhelmingly safe, it should be thought of first when there is mild muscle pain or discomfort.

Most home cupping sets are relatively easy to apply, and thanks to websites like Amazon, eBay, Wish.com and, Temu, you can have a set delivered to your door quickly and with little expense. If you wish, you can pick up other sets at your local Asian grocery store, many acupuncture clinics, and other wellness locations. Prices range depending on the type of cups, the number of cups included in the set, and any accessories that may be included. It's easy to get a budget-friendly kit that will last a long time with little maintenance.

The variety of sizes of these home cupping sets makes them quite versatile. Larger cups may not easily adhere to small areas on the body, so you will use smaller cups on your calves and arms, for example. Pulling out a few small cups and placing them on your calves is a great way to improve circulation and reduce muscle soreness after a run. Some kits sell cups in specialized shapes for body parts such as elbows and knees. I've never had much success using those as most cups adhere more easily to flatter, broader muscle groups.

Having a set of cups in your house will help you relieve all sorts of muscle pain, help with seasonal colds and chest congestion, and help with whole-body aches and unproductive coughs.

TERMS USED IN CUPPING

This book introduces you to the different types of cups available as well as a number of terms that describe the different cupping types, which you might hear when discussing cupping. Some of the terms overlap and are interchangeable, others have specific meanings that are particular to one system or refer to a specific technique. This book covers the two most common practices: static and sliding cupping.

The glossary below will help you if you find yourself talking with someone who receives or performs different styles of cupping. Healthcare professionals, such as licensed acupuncturists, use many of these techniques. If you are interested in experiencing these forms of cupping, search for a licensed professional in your area.

CUPPING GLOSSARY

DRY CUPPING: This term is interchangeable with static cupping but usually means "draws no blood." Some may take this to mean that there is no application of oils or lotion, but that isn't necessarily the case.

STATIC OR FIXED CUPPING: This term indicates that the cups are suctioned to the body and stay in place.

SLIDING OR MOVING CUPPING: For this method, a lubricant is first applied to the skin, then the cups. Once the cups attach, they glide across the area, providing both the benefits of cupping and a massage.

FLASH CUPPING: Using this technique doesn't necessarily produce bruising. Cups are applied and removed quickly across a large area. The idea is to increase circulation mildly in the region.

WET OR BLOOD CUPPING: This is a technique only someone with proper training should perform. "Wet" refers to blood being drawn by first pricking or cutting the skin. The theory is that blood cupping is more potent than regular cupping. Instead of bringing blood to the surface, the blood is physically removed from the body.

HIJAMA: This is the Muslim term for cupping—either wet or dry. In addition to having its own system of rules for how to apply the cups, *hijama* focuses on the spiritual aspects and includes principles of the Muslim faith, including applying cupping on specific holy days.

FIRE CUPPING: This term refers to the traditional way of adhering cups to the body by using fire to burn the oxygen out of the cups to create a vacuum. There are many techniques for doing this, but it is safest to leave it to professionals. You may also find a few grandmothers who are quite proficient in this technique.

Benefits of Cupping

Cupping at home allows you to provide yourself and your family relief from a slew of conditions. However, while it benefits many aches and pains, use good judgment when assessing health. With this in mind, please pay attention to this disclaimer.

Cupping does not replace medical care. You should consult medical professionals when there are severe conditions or when there is a lack of improvement of symptoms. Before trying cupping, talk to your primary care physician to make sure it is safe for you.

The number one reason people try cupping is for pain relief. Most of us experience neck and shoulder pain throughout our lives. The pain may come from injuries or accidents, but our modern sedentary lifestyle, long working hours, and lack of movement can be other culprits. A recent review of the literature[1] on cupping, which looks at all the high-quality medical studies, shows that cupping therapy is effective for upper and lower back pain. The pain does not need to be intense. It can simply be the result of overdoing it at the gym or the normal soreness after a long day at work. As I mentioned earlier, silicone cups are very portable, and some people keep a set in their gym bags and use them before or after a workout to loosen up muscle soreness or painful areas.

Cupping is beneficial for workout-related or injury-induced pain because it creates space. The suction pulls the skin away from the fascia—the connective tissue that covers the muscles and keeps the skin tightly attached. The fascia pulls away from the deeper muscle layers. The pull increases circulation to the tissue and creates space for inflammatory compounds like cytokines or lactic acid to move out, giving the muscles and joints some "room" to relax and alleviate the pain. A side effect of the suction is that the small capillaries at the surface break, leaving the body with the signature painless

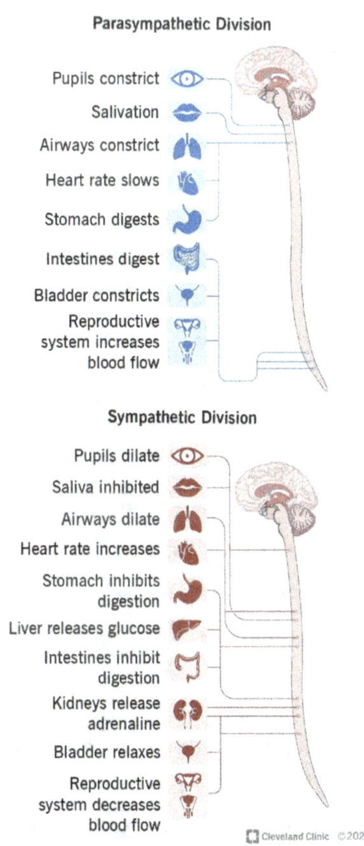

Autonomic Nervous System Functions

cupping bruises. These broken capillaries at the surface are not inert. They tell the body to keep fresh blood circulating through the surrounding areas for days while the bruise breaks down. The initial treatment starts the healing effect, and the marks continue for days afterward.

Cupping may have some mental health benefits as well, sparked by the whole-body effect of various types of bodywork. Our autonomic nervous system (ANS) is responsible for many of our body's functions without conscious thought. It has two different modes of operation: the sympathetic (fight or flight) and the parasympathetic (rest and digest). When stressed, anxious, or depressed, our body is often "stuck" in fight or flight mode. Our ANS is telling our bodies we are in danger and must concentrate on survival and not worry about how we feel emotionally.

Studies show that cupping helps switch our bodies back into the rest and digest stage of the ANS, allowing neurotransmitters—especially our "feel good" ones like serotonin, dopamine, and anandamide—to normalize, giving us peace of mind. This beneficial effect may be due to the body's response to its signals. When the ANS receives the "relaxation" signal, it kicks all of the "rest and digest" symptoms into action. For example, when cups are applied, they increase circulation locally and throughout the body. The signal tricks the body into thinking it is relaxed, causing all the other actions of the parasympathetic nervous system to activate, leading to a calmer, happier mind.

Another benefit of cupping, which has had prolonged historical use, is relief from chest congestion.[1] While we see people with antibiotic-resistant lung issues such as bronchitis or pneumonia in our clinic, these conditions should not be treated at home. A home practitioner should not attempt to treat anything more serious than mild chest congestion or cold and flu symptoms. If symptoms worsen, seek medical attention. Cupping can help the chest relax and open up, break up mucous, and help a cough become productive if the chest congestion is mild.

Now that we have an idea of how cupping can help us, let's look at the wide variety of home cupping styles available.

THE DIFFERENT STYLES OF CUPS FOR HOME USE

There are so many home cupping types and sets that it might seem overwhelming to choose. This book will introduce you to many different types and styles. In this chapter, we will discuss how they work, the individual pros and cons of each, and what to avoid. There are hundreds of brands available online, so while this book won't have every *brand*, we will cover every *style* of cup. If the cups you buy are not precisely the same color, size, or material, do not worry; they all function similarly and are easy to figure out. If you are trying to find the most cost-effective tools, I have included prices. Price ranges depend on the brand, the number of cups in the kit, and sometimes the quality of the set. You don't have to purchase a large set, but you may find you end up collecting many different types if you enjoy cupping.

Pumps (Sets range from $15 to $60.)

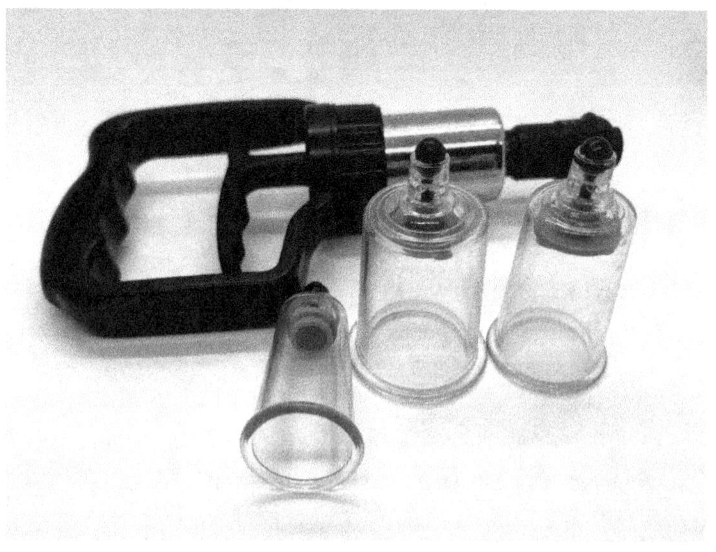

A Sample Pump Cupping Set

You will see some healthcare professionals using this style of cup. By far, it is the most common style—any larger Asian market will have a set or two on its shelves. The cups themselves are usually plastic with a one-way valve at the top. The kit will come with a hand pump that looks like a large syringe or a pistol. The end of the pump attaches to the one-way valve, and the vacuum occurs when pulling the trigger. Some pricier kits even come with a powered pump instead of a manual one.

Generally, pump-style cups are easy and fast to apply, and the pressure tends to be the strongest of all the different kinds of cups.

However, if you are using these kits on many people, I have doubts about the ability to clean them; the plastic valve at the top may hold bodily fluid even after washing. Also, because they are plastic, high heat or strong cleaning chemicals can cause the cups to become misshapen or can erode them. Therefore, these sets are best for non-clinical use and should be used only on friends and family.

Along with being available in Asian grocery stores, pump-style kits are abundant online and come in a wide variety of configurations, sizes, and shapes. Some come with travel cases and bonuses like *gua sha* (a scraping tool) or healing oil to allow for sliding cupping. Some oddly shaped cups may have a curved rim for application to areas of the body that are not flat, like elbows or knees. While these types of cups are suitable in theory, they are challenging to adhere to the body and tend to lose their seal with the slightest movements.

Some kits go a little too far. Search deep enough on the internet and you will stumble upon kits that contain pumps that—to put it as delicately as possible—are meant for breast, penis, and buttock enlargement. Please avoid these. Not only is there no evidence that they work, but placing cups on sensitive areas like these may cause harm. Although there isn't much documentation for this, there is concern that in highly vascular areas, larger blood vessels may rupture causing more bruising and possibly pain.

When shopping for a pump-style kit, there are some points to remember:

1. Some pump-style kits come with thin-walled glass cups. While they look nice, the thin wall is much more likely to crack, and the lip of the cup may chip. These chips and sharp edges could cut the skin. Usually, I recommend avoiding these sets unless you inspect the cups before applying them every time. In addition, these cups generally come with a significantly higher price tag and are more challenging to replace than the plastic versions if you

break one.

2. Not all kits are the same. You can buy additional cups separately, but you need to ensure that the pump from your set will fit on the valve of any cups you may purchase that were not part of the original kit.

3. Most pump-style kits suggest a maximum number of pumps to administer per cup. Each kit is different but the suggested number usually falls in the range of three to five pumps. Over-pumping the cups can be painful or cause blood blisters. So, keep the pressure mild to moderate and consistently tolerable.

Silicone (Sets range from $10 to $50.)

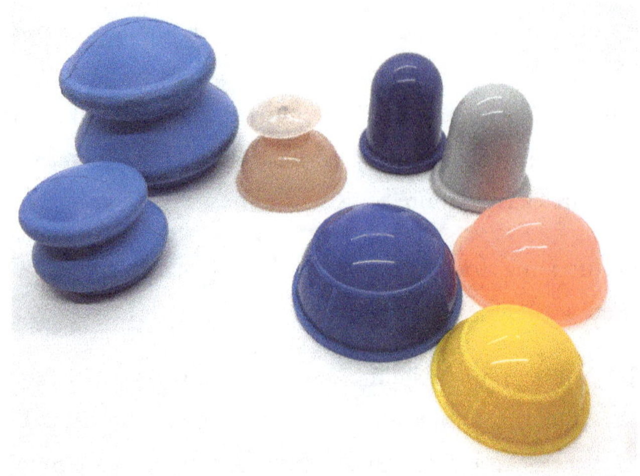

Examples of silicone cups

Silicone cups may be the next most widely available style. They can be any shape or size, so there is plenty of variety in this category. Some larger cups are manufactured with thick, firmer silicone and are appropriate for sliding techniques. Other silicone cups have a hard plastic handle on the top to allow sliding. The universal correlation between silicone cups is that you apply them by squeezing the air out of them as they sit on the body's surface.

When shopping for these kits, think about what size cups you want and how many. Larger cups are great but don't fit everywhere. Smaller cups fit everywhere, but you will need more to cover someone's hips or low back. Since these sets are relatively inexpensive and you can always mix them—buying a few different styles and experimenting is a good idea. My preferred cups for home use are readily available, portable, and inexpensive. My clinic sells a cupping kit containing 12 silicone cups that stack like a Russian nesting doll. The cups, when stacked together, are roughly the size of two halves of a tennis ball and can easily fit in a medicine cabinet, gym bag, or glove box. You can always have them readily available when you need them.

A NOTE ABOUT FACIAL CUPPING

Some cups with small openings and longer bodies are used for facial techniques. Facial cupping is done for cosmetic reasons and is a modern cupping adaptation. While it does work—and there are plenty of social media influencers promoting and demonstrating these techniques—this book will not discuss facial cupping because it can result in bruising. If you are interested in receiving facial cupping, it is best to seek a qualified professional—at least until you know what the sensation should feel like and how to avoid accidental bruising.

Bulbs (Prices range from $6 for a single to $30 for a full set.)

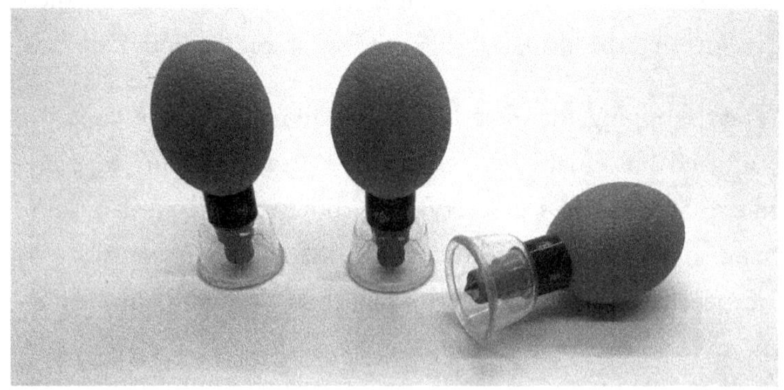

An Example of a Bulb Cupping Set

Bulb-style cups are a hybrid between the pump and silicone cups. The cup is usually plastic or glass with a silicone or rubber bulb at the top that is squeezed to create pressure. These cups also come in kits in several sizes. If they are glass, it's usually thin. This type of glass should always be inspected for chipping and damage before use.

Bulb-style cups are relatively easy to apply. Place the cup over the body part you wish to treat and squeeze the bulb. Many versions of this style of cup come with magnetic "pointers" in the middle. The idea behind a pointed magnet is for the patient to experience multiple therapies at the same time. Ideally, this cup style combines cupping therapy, acupressure, and magnet therapy all at once. To truly experience the benefits of all three, you need to know acupuncture points and magnetic therapy theory. Simply applying the cups to a sore area should still be beneficial, but it is hard to say how much of a synergistic effect might be noticed. Many kits have removable magnetic tips in them, allowing the user to choose whether to include the additional therapies.

Twisting Style (Usually sold in units of one to four, with a price range of $5 to $30.)

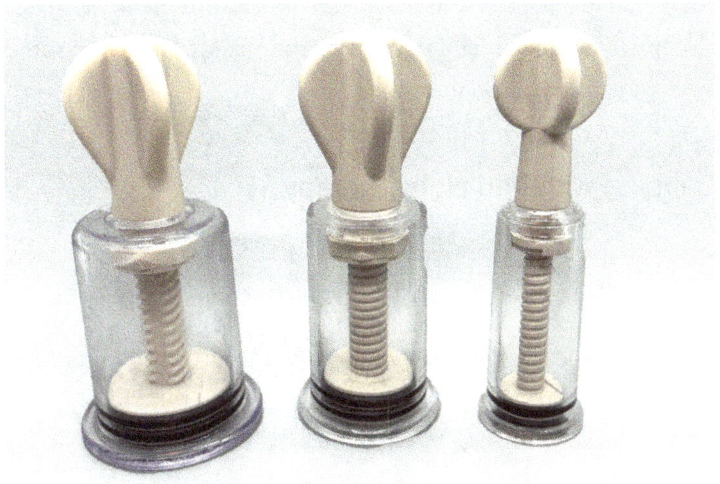

Examples of Twisting Cups

These cups tend to be a bit rarer. Instead of a large bulb at the top, they have a handle that looks a little like that on a pepper grinder. To achieve suction with these, the cup is applied to the skin and the handle is turned. The turning creates more space, causing the suction. These cups are attractive because they are less common and have more moving parts, but for those same reasons, they tend not to be used as much as the types previously discussed. Much like the pump-style cups, there are areas of the twisting-style cups that cannot easily be sterilized, which is a cause for concern for cleaning and sanitizing.

Combined Therapy and Novelty Cups (Prices for individual cups tend to range from $20 to $50.)

Combining modern and ancient therapies often yields unique treatments. It is exciting to see how the basic cupping technique has remained virtually the same for more than 4,000 years yet continues to evolve with different cultures and the advent of modern technologies. This section will discuss some of the newer styles of cups that add something extra to the therapy. Here are some modern takes on ancient medicine.

Cupping with Red Light Therapy

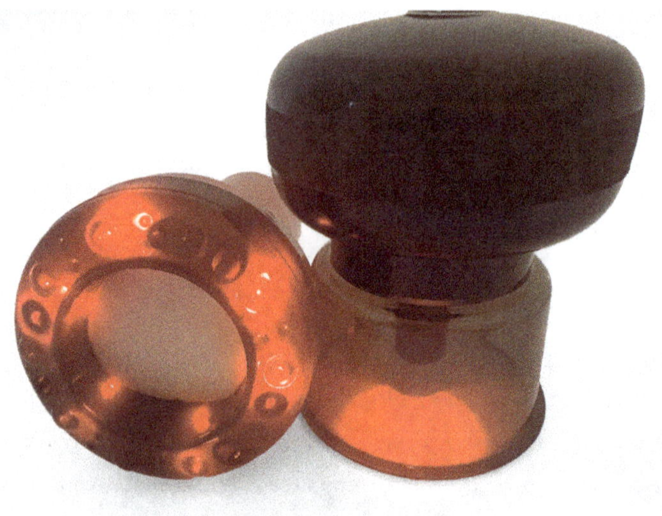

Examples of Red-Light Therapy Cups

Starting with one of the most novel combinations of cupping therapy and a "red hot" technology (pun shamelessly intended), these cups combine red light therapy with cupping. Red light therapy, or RLT, has been around for more than 40 years and falls into the category of photobiomodulation (PBM), which uses any frequency of light to change how the body functions. While several light colors have been researched, the red end of the spectrum—which includes visible red light, near-infrared light, and far-infrared light—has some therapeutic value. This end of the spectrum has been shown to increase circulation, help create more cellular energy, relieve pain, and produce collagen. All of these functions occur with cupping, and pairing the cupping with red light theoretically produces a synergistic effect.

These cups have a motorized pump to create the suction and several red LED lights to provide RLT. These innovations are exciting for practitioners like me, as my office is always trying to come up with therapeutic combinations—or stacks—to help people quickly and effectively recover from injury or illness.

When this style of cups first hit the scene, they were too expensive (more than $100) and too new (not many practitioners had experience with them yet) to take a chance on. Like every other style of cups, this style's value has been diluted by companies copying designs to make them cheaper, thus flooding the market. A quick search on Google yields prices between $39 and $199. While the cheaper prices may indicate lower quality items, the high-end price tags may not indicate the best tool. If you want to try RLT cups, it's probably best to aim for a price somewhere in the middle. If you are using Amazon, eBay, or any other site that provides reviews, make sure you read both the good and the bad before hitting the "Buy Now" button!

Vibrating Cups

This style of cup isn't very popular and may lead to scandalous results if typed into your search engine. These cups have some kind of motor that vibrates the cups after they adhere to the body. It isn't a flawed theory. Most of these cups have a silicone base and a battery-operated motor located at the top. There are professional techniques in which the cups are placed and shaken when activated to move the tissue more. Some of these cups are relatively cheap but harder to find. If you want to try something a little "out there," this type of cup may fit the bill.

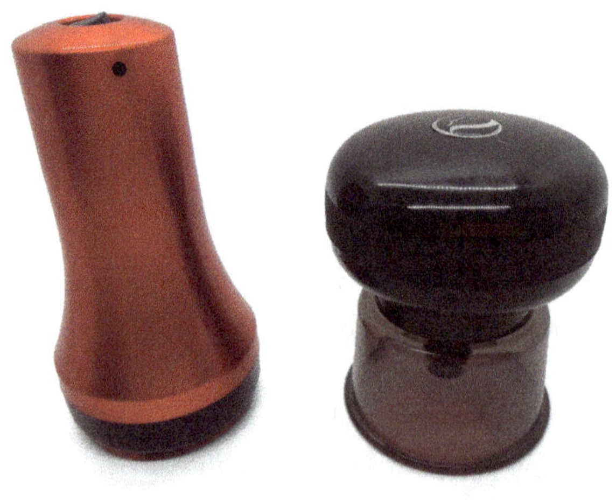

Different Styles of Vibrating Cups

Cupping, Gua Sha, Heating

This is another multiple-intervention style of cups—a modern attempt to combine multiple therapies. *Gua sha* is a fantastic technique that has been appropriated and called Graston's technique or Instrument Assisted Soft Tissue Mobilization (IASTM). The name *gua sha* translates to "Scraping Sand," and when done correctly should leave lines of "bruising" along the length of the treated muscles. It is excellent for pain and can be done as a standalone therapy. These cups use a battery-operated pump to create the suction and have a built-in heating element. They are designed to slide across muscle groups, providing a more extensive treatment area. Technically, this isn't *gua sha*. It is a technique called sliding cupping, which will be discussed in the upcoming chapters. I have tried out several of these styles of cups from different online stores and, sadly, haven't been that impressed. The concept is excellent, and when the cups were suctioned, they felt good, but I found they often slipped while sliding and weren't easy to operate. The heating elements were not adjustable and didn't add much to the treatment.

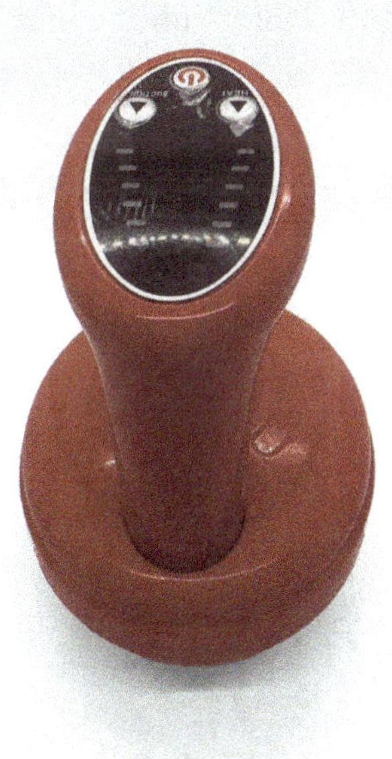

A Combination Gua Sha Cup

TENS (Transcutaneous Electrical Nerve Stimulation)

TENS units provide electrical stimulation to a muscle group in an attempt to reduce pain, release tightness, and improve circulation. There was a time when these units were bigger and only found in health offices that worked with injuries and recovery. Now many units are available online, are smaller than a phone, and can even be charged with a USB. The TENS units come with cables that attach to sticky pads that go over a painful area. When the machine is turned on, the electrical current can be turned up until the person wearing it gets some relief. Adding cupping to this device should increase circulation in the area. Instead of using sticky pads, this style of cup has an electrically conductive rim and a port for attaching the TENS unit cable. To use these cups, you will need a TENS unit, specialized cords to plug into the cups (the cords are not always included with the unit), and a conductive gel to apply around the rim of the cup. You won't feel the current without the gel. I have not seen a kit where everything is included, but all of these individual items are available online and are relatively inexpensive.

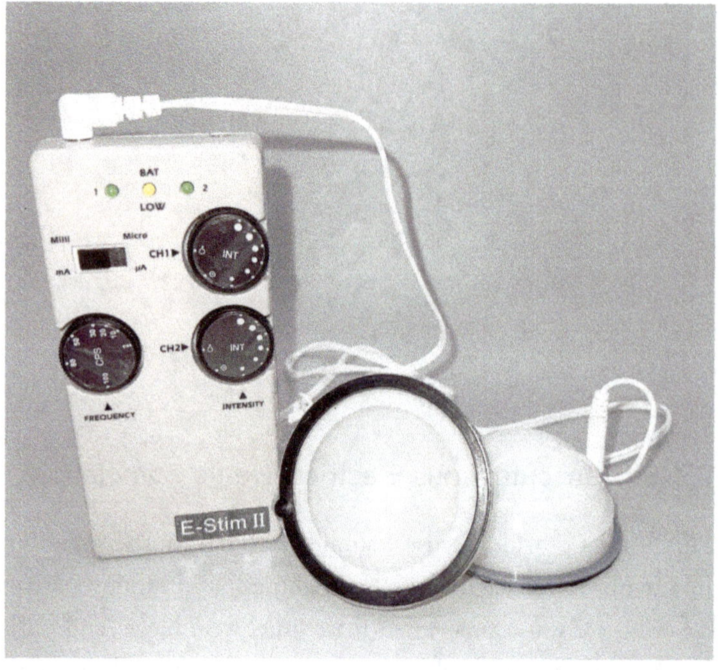

Sample TENS Cups

Novelty Shapes (Heart-shaped sets range from $20 to $80.)

Examples of Novelty Cups

As I mentioned earlier in the history section, another acupuncturist beat me to this idea. Now you can find cups shaped like hearts and stars and, soon enough I'm sure, there will be other shapes. Most of these are made of silicone or are the plastic pump variety. If nothing else, these cups are fun. While they do work, they are designed more to leave a shape than to cover an area. Even though there are more people aware of cupping today than when I started in the field, someone will always stare or comment when they spot cupping marks on a person. If you want to make your cupping marks a "statement piece," try some of these fancy-shaped cups and you will surely get all the looks!

Fire Cupping

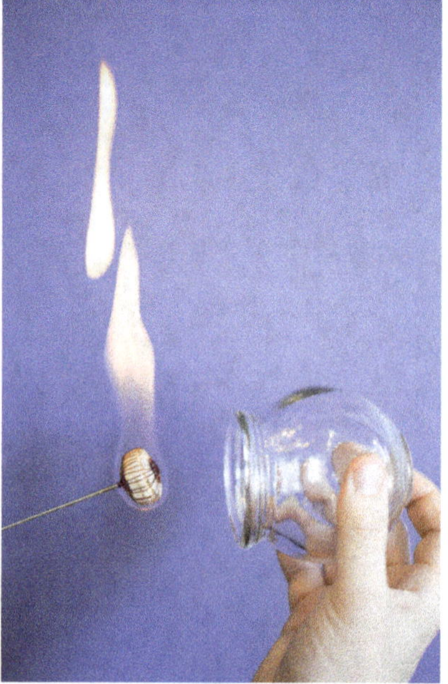

Fire Cupping

While plenty of grandmothers out there did fire cupping in their kitchen, I'm going to advise that people leave this to professionals. Yes, there is a bit more showmanship with fire cupping, and it just "looks cooler," but in addition to the risk of starting an unintentional fire, there is also a risk to the person receiving the cupping. If you're trying to do this to yourself, it is extremely risky. Even if you are working on someone else, please beware. People who aren't adequately trained have often burned someone by heating up the cups. The cups should never get hot and the fire is merely another way to remove the oxygen and create a vacuum. With such a large number of safe cupping options available, leave this one alone.

CUPPING RULES, CONSIDERATIONS, AND CONTRAINDICATIONS

"Prepare and prevent, don't repair and repent."

—AUTHOR UNKNOWN

Cupping therapy is very safe, especially when we remove fire from the equation. This section will explore the rules of cupping, which should serve as guidelines for when, how long, and why to cup. Most importantly, it is necessary to understand when to use caution and when cupping is inappropriate. Even the safest modalities are not risk-free, so read this section carefully to ensure you have the best possible experience with cupping therapy. I will highlight any red flags or problems that you should definitely avoid. Once again, please do not mistake home cupping therapy for medical treatment, and if the condition seems too severe or sounds like a red flag, seek a licensed medical practitioner before performing cupping.

THE BASIC GUIDELINES:

When to Use Cups

1. Muscle Soreness

This is the perfect instance for cupping. In general, find indurations or adhesions—fancy ways to say "knots"—and try to cover them with the cups. Whether muscle soreness is pain from physical labor or an intense workout, cupping can be a perfect fit. In a later chapter, I'll show you some photos as inspiration.

2. Chest Congestion

There are two areas that can be cupped for chest congestion. The front of the chest can help break up mucous and make coughing more productive. For women, make sure you work above the breast tissue. On the back, working in the areas of the shoulders and down between the shoulder blades can help break up phlegm and allow for deeper breathing.

3. Stress

Cupping is one of the many physical modalities that can trigger your parasympathetic nervous system to switch on. Your parasympathetic is often referred to as your rest and digest mode. Switching into this part of the autonomic nervous system leads to better circulation, deeper breathing, and balancing of feel-good neurotransmitters like serotonin and dopamine. If you think about the tightness that occurs when you are under stress, these are the areas you want to treat. Believe it or not, many people get cupping because they enjoy it. This is a valid reason for cupping, so long as there are no underlying red flags.

Amount of Time to Retain Cups

The duration of a cup's application is usually five to 20 minutes per area. Some people will work on one section of the body for that time and then move to another area. The session itself may last much longer this way. For example, cups are applied to the shoulder for 10 minutes, then the upper back for 10 minutes, then the lower back for 10 minutes.

There are some factors that determine the length of time to keep the cups on a spot. First is comfort; the person receiving cupping should feel mild-to-moderate pressure. With silicone-style cups, this is pretty easy to achieve. Pump, bulb, and twist styles can be pushed past this level, which you should avoid. If the cup is uncomfortable, take it off and re-apply it more lightly.

Another essential factor in retaining cups is the color beneath the cup rims. The textbook color would be a reddish-purplish mark, and that would indicate that the spot is "done." The mark may contain small red or purple dots called purpura or petechia. If you are nearing the 20-minute timeframe and do not see redness, remove the cups anyway; not every area of the body has the same number of capillaries, and some areas—based on body composition—may not turn red at all. This is why many people prefer clear cups, so they can visually determine the redness before removing the cups. If you use opaque cups, you can remove one to check and re-apply it if it hasn't been in place long enough.

Leaving cups in place too long or applied too strongly runs the risk of causing blood blisters and pain. While that condition isn't immediately dangerous, it doesn't feel good and could lead to infection. If this occurs, clean and dress the area with sterile gauze and use an antibiotic cream if possible. Do not cup that area again until the blisters completely heal. This side effect is rare, but it is essential to know how to deal with it.

Frequency of Cupping

The frequency at which you apply cups is also dependent on several factors. Some people will say weekly, but if you are repeating in the same areas and bruising from the previous round has not largely resolved, you need to wait. If the cupping marks are lighter but not completely resolved, you can cup again—just retain them for a shorter amount of time.

If you wish to do cupping more frequently, use different locations for the cups. Simply avoid any dark cupping marks.

There is the option to apply cups very lightly and not allow a bruise to set up. With this method, you can cup the same area more than once a week, but this technique does not give you the same results as one more vigorous session. Sensitive people may prefer this, which is an excellent option to keep in the back of your mind. In this case, you may lightly apply the cups, monitoring and removing the cups at the first sign of bruising. If you have opaque cups and can't see the color change, apply them for two to three minutes and then check.

Pain While Cupping

Strong cupping may be intense and slightly uncomfortable, but in no way should it be painful. If the cups are too strong, you risk tissue damage. Remember that you can apply the cups gently and leave them in place longer to achieve the same results. This is a no-pain, no-gain situation. Sometimes you can "burp" the cups to alleviate pressure by pressing your finger under the edge of the cup. If you do this right, you can get a controlled reduction in pressure. More often than not, the seal is broken, and the cup detaches. With these cupping methods, it's quick and easy to re-apply them with less pressure.

Make Sure the Cup Fits the Area

Cups attach best to broad muscles that are relatively flat. Today's silicone cups come in so many sizes that you can fit cups on forearms and calves, which is excellent. Choose smaller cups for small areas and wider cups for broader areas. It's relatively intuitive. If you only have a kit with one size, you may need to skip some spots.

Maximum Pressure on Pump-Style Cups

Usually, cups for home use have an upper limit on how strong the vacuum can get. Feedback from the "cup-ee" is critical. Pump-style cups have an exception: the one-way valve allows for intense pressure to occur quickly. Most kits recommend a maximum number of pumps. The number varies from kit to kit but is usually three to five pumps per cup. Keep this in mind when using this style of cup. Most of these kits come out of Asia and may not have directions you can read. In that case, aim for three pumps maximum for each cup, but stop if it feels too intense. The number of pumps can and will vary from person to person and even locations on the same person, so there's no need to keep the same strength at every site.

SPECIAL CONSIDERATIONS:

Areas with Excessive Body Hair

Body hair is natural, but when you are counting on a smooth lip of a cup to make a seal against the skin, body hair can get in the way. You do not need to shave the areas to get the cups to stick. There is an easier way. Using oil or one of the many topical formulas discussed in the next chapter can not only help with the hairy situation but possibly elevate the whole cupping experience.

People Who Bruise Easily

Bruising easily isn't a contraindication for cupping, but you should make sure that you are watching the cups closely and either using less suction or leaving the cups on for a shorter time. You may also need to reduce the frequency of cupping sessions to allow the bruises to clear entirely before applying them again. If you or someone you want to try cupping on falls into this category, just make sure there is no clotting issue and be extra careful.

People Who Have Many Superficial Veins

This is another situation where cupping isn't contraindicated, but you should avoid more prominent veins and anything that is raised or painful to the touch. For any vascular conditions like deep vein thrombosis or any issue where the vasculature may rupture, cupping should not be performed. That statement will be reiterated in the red flags section ahead.

Spider and varicose veins often occur in the legs when we age, and our vessels lose elasticity. In most cases, there shouldn't be any issues with cupping areas that do not have visible veins. If there are only one or two small visible veins on a hamstring, you can still cup the hamstring but avoid doing so directly over the vein.

People Who Do Not Like Strong Stimulation

Cupping should "fit" the person's body and constitution. If a person is robust, muscular, and healthy overall, they may tolerate and enjoy strong cupping. If someone is frail or very sensitive, milder cupping should be applied. This counts not only for the strength with which each cup is applied but also for the number of areas cupped and the duration of treatment if you are cupping yourself. If you are cupping someone else, make sure you promote feedback throughout the process.

People Who May Be Embarrassed by the Marks

If you picked up this book, you probably expect perfectly circular marks that let everyone know you have been cupped. If the marks are going to be visible, you will get some looks and comments—usually some overused reference to an octopus. People in the know may ask you where you got treatment or why you picked that place. It can be an excellent conversation starter. In my clinic, I call the marks "walking advertisements," especially in the warm months when people wear shorts and tank tops.

If you are going to cup someone else, make sure they are aware of the bruising. You don't need your friend calling you screaming about the expensive dress they can't wear to a fancy outing due to the visible marks up and down their back. A colleague of mine had an angry phone call from an angry husband who'd "spent too much money on a dress to have his wife look all beat up like that." His wife, however, felt marked relief after the session and didn't mind the attention at the event at all. If you are cupping on yourself, at this point, you should be expecting marks. Just make sure that whoever else you try it on is well aware of the process and outcome.

RED FLAGS, DO NOT CUP

Pregnancy

While, yes, people do get cupping during pregnancy, it's best to avoid cupping while pregnant unless it's performed by a licensed healthcare professional. There are no studies on cupping therapy and its safety during pregnancy. This doesn't mean that cupping will cause problems. However, there are some reasons to avoid cupping at this time. It is a sad fact that roughly 30 percent of all pregnancies don't make it to term, according to the March of Dimes. Many of these miscarriages happen after what appears to be a perfectly healthy start of a pregnancy, when even the most advanced testing does not reveal a problem. Then, if someone tries a new activity or treatment and there is a spontaneous miscarriage, that new activity is often blamed even if it is entirely unrelated, and even when the session may have been done weeks before the miscarriage.

According to Chinese medicine, a fetus is an accumulation of qi, (or life force) and blood[2], which is why we want those substances to stay in place. Cupping therapy vigorously moves the qi and blood. Some practitioners may argue that it only moves these substances locally, directly under the area of the cup, so treating the upper back, arms, and legs should be okay during pregnancy.

However, when there are other treatments for pregnant women that we know to be safe, why take the risk?

Open Wounds

While in acupuncture school, I learned the expression, "Don't spank a crying baby." This phrase fits well when it comes to cupping and open wounds. Avoid cuts, scrapes, and anything that may be bleeding or oozing on the skin's surface when applying cups. Areas with acne may benefit from cupping, but there is a good chance that the cups might extract oils, blood, and puss from the skin if you do this.

You may see specialized kits for bug bites that include tiny cups to help draw out the venom. However, bug bite kits are specialized cups with mixed reviews.

Skin Conditions

Even if there isn't a visible open wound, you should make sure that the skin is clear in the area you are applying cups. Eczema and psoriasis are two of the most common skin conditions, and you can see areas of dryness, cracking, scaling, and, in extreme cases, oozing of the skin. Some may think we should "draw out the toxins" from the affected area. Please DO NOT do this. You can make the area worse by causing tissue damage or an infection. You can, however, cup safely on a person who has skin conditions if you pick an area that has no issues. Make sure you stay far away from any abnormal skin texture or lesions.

Hemophilia, Blood Thinners, and Clotting Disorders

I have been in practice for more than two decades and have not once had a true hemophiliac come in for cupping or acupuncture. It's not that they don't exist, it's more likely that they know enough about themselves and the treatments I provide to know that it may not be worth the risk. If someone does have hemophilia or a clotting disorder, DO NOT perform cupping on them. The risk is not worth the reward.

The use of cupping on people taking blood thinners is questionable. Always err on the side of caution. I know licensed practitioners who do cupping on people taking low-dose aspirin and prescription blood thinners. For the home user, this is a risk you should not take.

IMPORTANT TAKEAWAYS

- When cups are applied, they should be at a moderate pressure, not too painful

- They may be left on for 10 to 15 minutes or until the area becomes dark red/ purple; you may see some purpura or petechia forming. This is a good sign, but cupping should stop when this occurs

- People with excessive body hair may need to be coated with a NON-FLAMMABLE oil or cream

- Cups will adhere to flat areas better than curves. Smaller cups may be necessary to get into the neck or joints

RED FLAGS — DO NOT PERFORM CUPPING

- During pregnancy

- On open wounds

- On anyone with hemophilia and other clotting disorders

- Directly on skin conditions

OILS, LINIMENTS, AND CREAMS: UPGRADING YOUR CUPPING

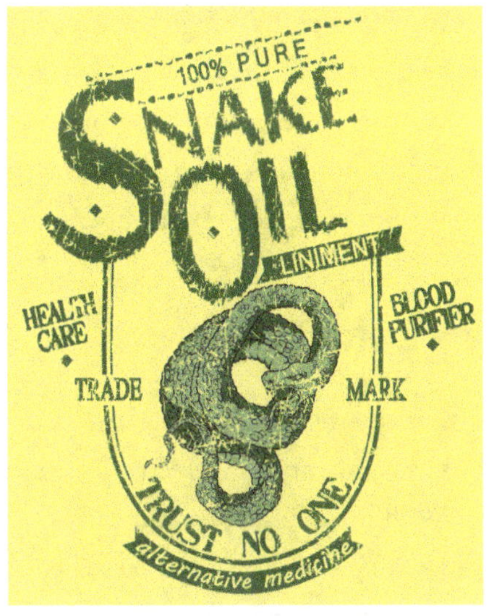

Not all oils are appropriate for cupping

There are several reasons to apply something topical before you start cupping. Body hair is one area of concern that we discussed in the previous section. Applying a lubricant can help solve this problem by matting the hair against the skin to create a smooth surface. On smooth skin, lubricants can make the cupping more intense, and on hairy parts of the body, they can help keep the cups from losing suction.

Static cupping, where the cups are not moved, can be done without any topical compound applied, but a lubricant is needed for sliding cupping or it will be pretty painful. Some people also prefer to use a topical compound even for static cupping. One major reason to do this is to add more relief to the session. Herbs and aromatic essential oils can be used to help relax muscles, relieve pain, and open up the airways. All of these are great reasons to add a topical formula.

There are so many possibilities when choosing to apply a compound to the skin before performing cupping. Many of today's formulas also have herbs to enhance pain relief or help break up congestion. We will start with some oils you may already have in your kitchen and then discuss some commonly used liniments available online or from your local Asian supermarket.

FROM YOUR PANTRY

Let's start with what you might already have in your kitchen. Natural oils like olive, coconut, and grapeseed oil all work well. A little goes a long way. With these oils, you want to keep a thin layer on the area you are working on; there is no reason to apply so much that it drips. Avoid heavily processed vegetable oils or anything that may go on thickly. A good rule of thumb is that if it's considered healthy to eat, it is acceptable to use for cupping.*

Be careful with nut oils. Yes, most nut oils are healthy. However, given that nut allergies can be serious, it is best to make sure whoever is using the oil is not allergic to it.

FROM YOUR MEDICINE CABINET

While I'm not a fan of petroleum-based oils, I have seen a good amount of Vaseline or Vicks VapoRub used in some clinics and households. They get the job done, and the menthol and camphor in the VapoRub can help break up congestion in the chest and are topical analgesics for some pain relief. Today, there are many plant-based products that are thick like Vaseline but are not made from petroleum. While these thick products are not my personal preference, they can be used, and remember, a little goes a long way. They will not absorb into the skin like lighter oils, so be prepared to clean them off the skin when you are done cupping.

FROM YOUR LOCAL PHARMACY

Tiger Balm

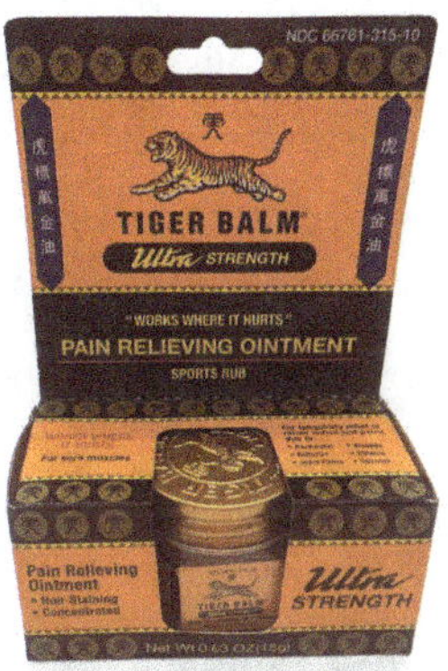

Tiger Balm

Tiger Balm became widely popular in the U.S. in the 1990s. Initially from Singapore, this iconic formula never caught on in mainland China. When the company had a problem marketing to

Asians who associated the smell with their grandparents using it as a cure-all, the company decided to look to the West and began a marketing campaign that included Joe Montana and Jerry Rice and landed their product on the shelves of every major pharmacy in the USA.

While I personally prefer other products for cupping, Tiger Balm's blend of herbs and aromatics provides solid pain relief, breaks up congestion, and is even reported to help with digestive issues. (Use it topically only, do not ingest!)

In addition to camphor and menthol, which offer strong sinus-clearing effects and pain relief (and are standard in every similar product) Tiger Balm also contains capsaicin: The compound that puts the heat in hot peppers causes blood vessels to open, bringing fresh blood to the cupping area, and clearing out inflammation. Methyl salicylate, another ingredient, functions in a similar fashion to aspirin—reducing inflammation and relieving pain—and a blend of essential oils is reported to reduce pain and round out Tiger Balm's distinct smell. This widely available product works well and many people already have it sitting in the medicine cabinet. It's a great choice if you are looking for pain relief or to break up congestion while doing cupping.

Biofreeze

Biofreeze is another topical formula that, at one point, was only available for professional use. It is now readily available for consumers in the pain-relief aisle of every pharmacy. In addition to its gel form, which is preferred for cupping, Biofreeze is also available with a roll-on applicator and as a spray. Those two types are okay to apply before static cupping. For sliding cupping, the gel beneficially provides the right amount of glide to help the cups move smoothly while keeping the right amount of friction.

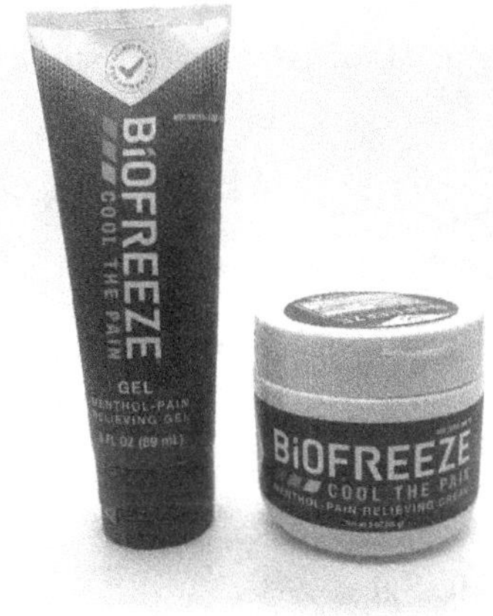

Biofreeze

Overall, Biofreeze is safe and does provide some pain relief. It's very similar to the old-school BENGAY or Aspercreme.

One unique thing that Biofreeze adds to its mix of ingredients is *Ilex paraguariensis*, which sounds like a fancy herb, but is actually none other than Argentina's favorite caffeinated beverage, yerba mate. While Biofreeze's marketing mentions Ilex, it does not say why it is used. The results of one study by the National Center for Biotechnology Information suggests that "the intake of mate extract has potential as a treatment for both postoperative pain and neuropathic pain." [3]

Either way, Biofreeze is a popular option for topical pain relief and can be purchased anywhere that you can buy pain-relief medicines.

Massage Creams and Oils

Many massage oils and creams are available for professional massage therapists and for home use. These products are intended to go on the skin and should work for cupping. If you have a favorite brand, feel free to use it. While there are far too many to list, here are some general categories of massage oils that you may want to try:

- **Hypoallergenic**
  These oils are specifically designed for sensitive skin. If you or the person you are working on reacts to certain chemicals, perfumes, or other compounds found in skincare products, look for hypoallergenic oils.

- **Medicated/Herbal**
  These oils and creams have compounds added for their therapeutic properties—mainly in the realm of pain relief or inflammation reduction. Many could be considered a "professional grade" menthol-and-camphor blend that you can pick up anywhere. Some will have single herbs to help alleviate pain or loosen muscles.

- **Essential Oil Infused**
  Essential oils have lovely smells that are claimed to help a wide array of symptoms. Some products are made with essential oils in them, and some are unscented carriers into which you can drop single oils or a blend of your own. Adding essential oils to a treatment provides both topical help and a pleasant scent.

Readily Available Traditional Chinese Medicine (TCM) Ointments and Oils

Whether or not the Chinese invented cupping, they have been

performing it within the realm of Chinese medicine for more than 2,000 years. Cupping therapy is often grouped with acupuncture, moxibustion, and *gua sha* as a modality that may be performed during an acupuncture treatment. This long-standing use by TCM practitioners and Asian households has yielded techniques and theories for cupping that differ from the approaches to treatment in other regions of the world.

In China, people use thousands of topical formulas for pain relief and often combine them in cupping therapy. This is partially due to the country's sheer size; it made more sense for people in one area of the country to create their own formulas rather than have them shipped in from somewhere else. It is also due to the vast volume of herbal knowledge that the Chinese—and Asia as a whole—have compiled. This led to the compilation of a *Materia Medica*, or book of medicinal herbs, which catalogs thousands of herbs and discusses uses, preparations, safety, dosage, and even what other herbs to combine to mitigate side effects and improve outcomes.

Combining the traditional benefits of cupping with the sophisticated knowledge of Chinese herbal medicine can add a significant synergistic effect to your treatments. TCM oils and ointments make up another category of topical formulas that is far too broad to cover here. Below, are descriptions of the most commonly available TCM oils in the U.S. They can often be found at your local acupuncturist's office and some larger Asian grocery stores.

If you have an acupuncturist or auntie in Asia with a favorite TCM oil, you might use what they recommend. If you have difficulty finding TCM oils, a simple search on Amazon will get most of the selections listed below to your door within two days.

I've included pictures for each product. I recommend that you try to make sure that what you order looks like the image I've provided here. There are knock-offs of many famous formulas, and the name and packaging may be similar. In many cases, these companies cut corners by reducing the concentration of herbs, using lower-quality ingredients, or simply not including them at all. Some copycats even include pharmaceutical ingredients. The formulas included in this text are recognizable, and in most cases, fakes are apparent.

Dit Da Wan Hua Oil

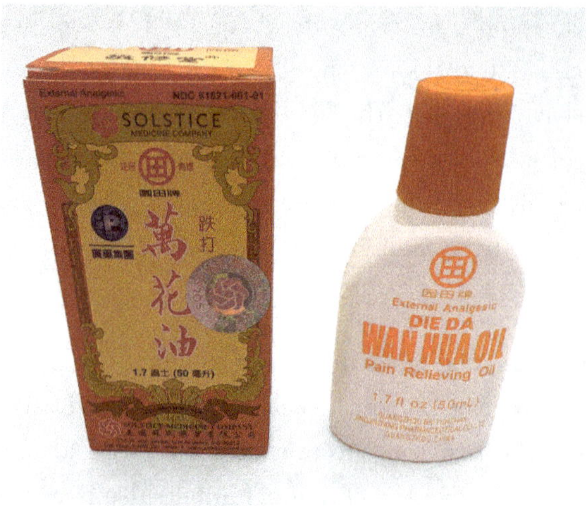

Dit Da Wan Hua

If you were to walk into most acupuncture colleges across the U.S., *Dit Da Wan Hua* oil is most likely the standard oil you would find used for sliding cupping in their student clinics. *Dit Da* means "fall, hit," and as the name sounds, this herbal formula is used for traumatic injuries but is also a good help for chronic pain and muscle aches. Sometimes noted as "Traumatic Injury Ten-Thousand Flowers Oil" in English, this herbal formula also helps with chronic pain and muscle aches. (While its list of aromatic and floral ingredients is long, a thousand may be an overstatement!) This topical herbal formula is the only true oil in this section and is mild enough that most people enjoy using it. It isn't the most potent formula for injuries but is readily available and used in our clinics. Being an oil, a little goes a long way, and a thin layer on the cupped area helps the cups adhere and provides enough glide to help get the proper amount of friction when sliding the cups. Because other topicals are quickly absorbed, many practitioners put this on the patient as a second layer or mix it with another formula to find the right ratio of adherence and slide. This oil is versatile and can be used for massage and *gua sha* therapy.

"White" Oils

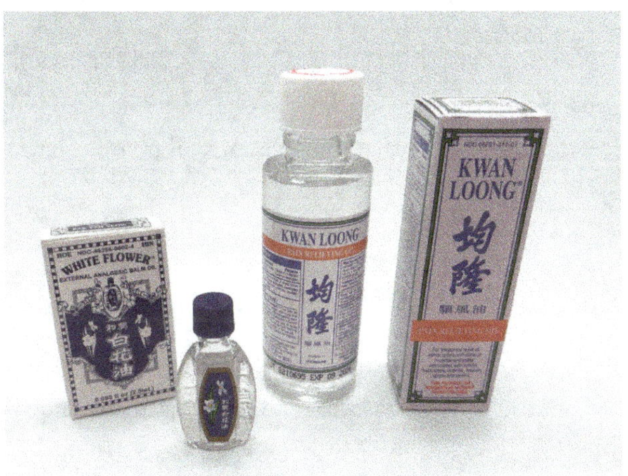

"White" Oils

Many "white oils" are used in traditional Chinese medicine. These oils are clear, not white, and they usually contain camphor and menthol and have that distinctive "I'm sore" smell. Many contain other essential oils that help open the sinuses and relieve pain. One of the ingredients I look for is methyl silicate, which is also found in Tiger Balm. Clear liniments like these are considered to have a cooling nature and are best applied to warm and slightly swollen areas. This compound adds relief to swelling, with effects that are very similar to those of aspirin. The most commonly available are Kwan Loong and White Flower oil.

In addition to being widely available, white oils tend to be relatively low cost. Buying a bottle of several different brands to see which one you like best won't cost much. You can also use them as a normal pain liniment without cupping. People often put a few drops on a handkerchief to sniff occasionally when their sinuses are acting up. They also put a drop or two on bug bites to help with the itching and pain. Almost all of the brands come in different sizes, including some tiny bottles that you can keep in your pocket, just in case.

These oils absorb quickly so they are okay for static cupping but may need to be mixed with a more viscous oil if you want to slide the cups.

Wood Lock or Wong To Yick

This one is a personal favorite. In addition to the usual menthol, camphor, and methyl salicylate, it contains lavender and wintergreen oils. It is "cooling" by nature and also has a delightful smell. This brand had production issues for a while and was very hard to get for a few years prior to COVID-19. Look for the photo of the dapper man on the bottle. There are a few knock-offs of this formula, which aren't that bad either, but I prefer to go with the one that has been around for a long time. This liniment absorbs quickly, so it should be mixed with oil if you intend to slide the cups.

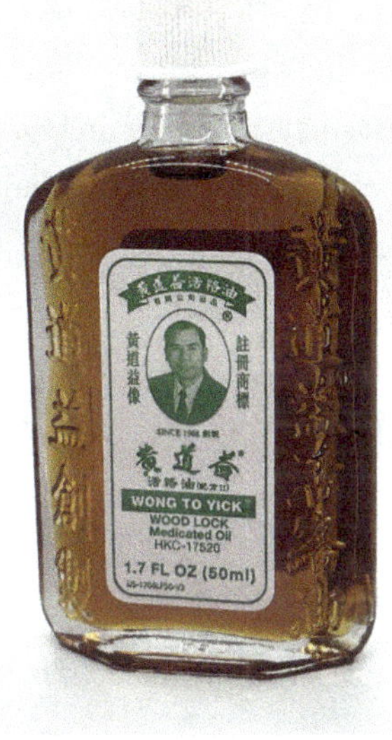

Wood Lock Oil

Red Oils

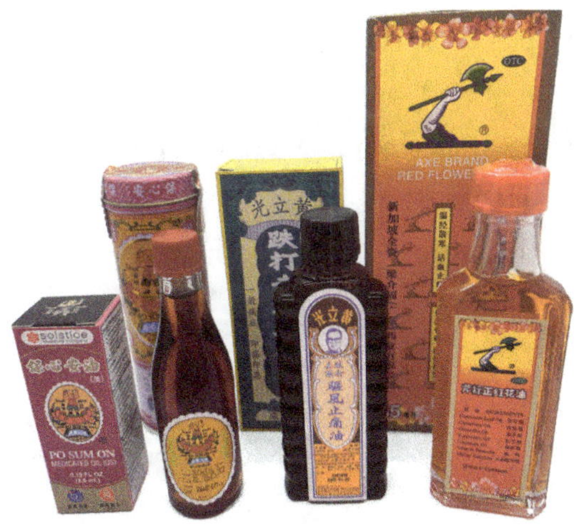

"Red" Oils

Hong Hua, or Red Flower oil and *Po Sum On*, or peaceful heart oil, are two of the most common of this TCM category. Many people enjoy these not only for their pleasant smell but also because *Po Sum On* sounds like "pour some on" in English. Red oils have the same basic formula as the white oils but include cinnamon and other herbs and spices that add warming properties to the oil. These formulas are great when people have a cold, stiff joints, or generally prefer heat to cold.

IMPORTANT TAKEAWAYS

- Oils, creams, and liniments can benefit your cupping.

- Some kind of lubricant is necessary for sliding cupping.

- There are a wide variety of products available from many different sources.

- Pick a product that has properties that align with what you are trying to accomplish with cupping.

- Make sure the product you choose won't irritate the person's skin.

- Be wary of knockoffs.

- Be careful to avoid open wounds, skin eruptions, and cuts.

STATIC CUPPING

The following two chapters will introduce static and sliding cupping and explain how each type of cup can be applied. We will discuss the areas where the cups are placed in the section afterward. Within a short period, you should feel comfortable applying and removing cups.

Every style of cup previously mentioned can be used for static cupping. Static, or fixed, cupping is the most common form of cupping worldwide and has been throughout history. The cups are applied and left alone until it is time to remove them.

Here is a step-by-step guide to static cupping, including how to attach and remove each type of cup:

1. *Choose an Area*

Choosing the areas to cup is an essential part of the process. When choosing an area based on pain, it is crucial to ensure that the cups can be comfortably applied. Cupping effects can extend beyond the rim of the cups, so there is some leeway. Look at the entire area and try to include muscles associated with the affected area.

If you are cupping to support the lungs, look at areas on the upper back, shoulders, and chest. Stay away from breast tissue.

In general, applying the cups to wider, broader muscles makes it easier to get suction. Making sure that a cup will fit within the muscle on which you are applying it will also help achieve stronger suction.

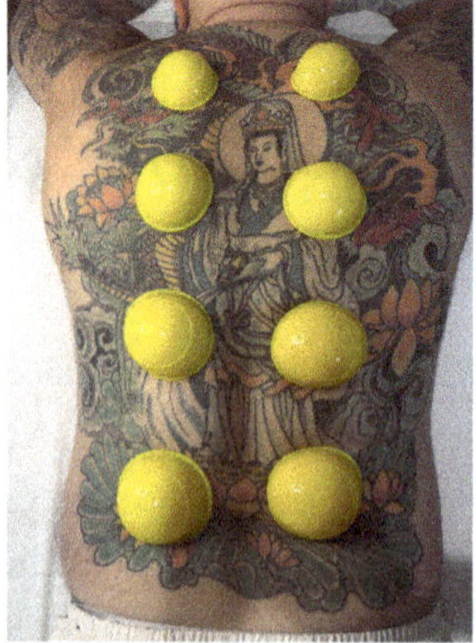

Possible Areas to Treat on the Back

Before applying the cups, look at the skin and determine if you wish to use a topical oil or liniment. As we previously discussed, adding something topically can enhance the treatment but may not be necessary. Oil will make the process easier if the area has body hair. Apply enough to leave a thin coat; it does not need to be dripping. Specific topical formulas will absorb quickly and may require you to work quickly or apply more when changing the placement of the cups.

2. *Attach and Remove the Cups*

The different cup types use the same principle for attachment; they remove some air from the space inside the chamber formed between the cup and the skin. This creates a vacuum and draws the skin up into the cup. While each style of cup removes the air differently, all of them should be applied with moderate pressure. Some may feel more intense than others, but none of them should be painful or make the person being treated feel that they need to suffer through the experience. Remember, you can attach the cups with less pressure and leave them in place a little longer to avoid creating pain.

Removing the cups is another important part of the treatment. While each style of cup has its own style of removal, all of them require releasing the vacuum. Do not try to simply use force to pull the cup off the area being treated. You may be successful if the cup is attached lightly, but in most cases this will cause pain and possible injury to the person being treated. When in doubt, press down on the skin and slip your finger under the lip of the cup. This will break the seal and release the cup without discomfort. It also yields a distinct popping sound.

   a.   Pumps

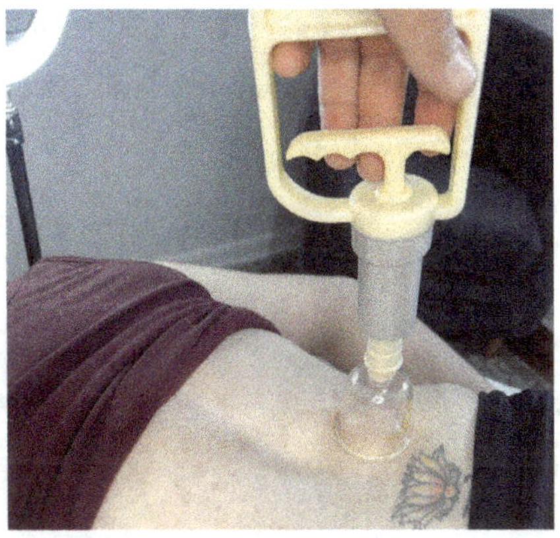

Pump Style Cup Being Applied

To apply this style of cup, place the cup on the body in a location you want to treat. Place the pump opening (opposite the trigger) over the cup and pump. Make sure you don't over pump, and if you can't find or read the instructions, do not pump the trigger more than three to five times.

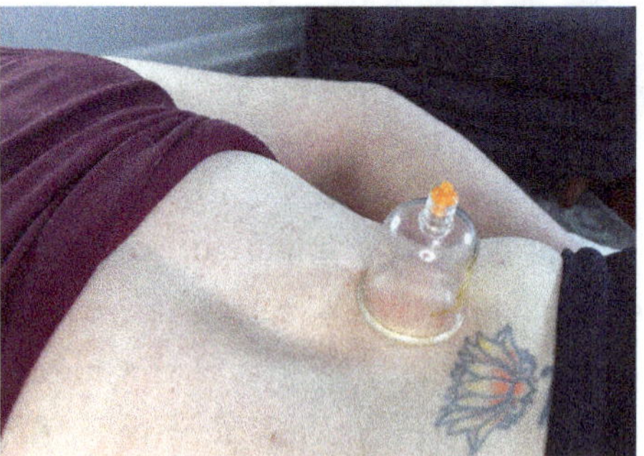

Pump Style Cup Adhered to Skin

After the treatment, there are two ways to remove this type of cup. You can remove the cups by pressing down and sliding a finger under the lip of the cup where it meets the skin. If the cup is very tight, this may be difficult. This is often the least comfortable part of the treatment, though it is still tolerable. The other method is to pull up the small stem that comes out of the valve at the top of the cup. Both methods should release the vacuum and you will hear a sound letting you know the seal is broken and the cup can be removed.

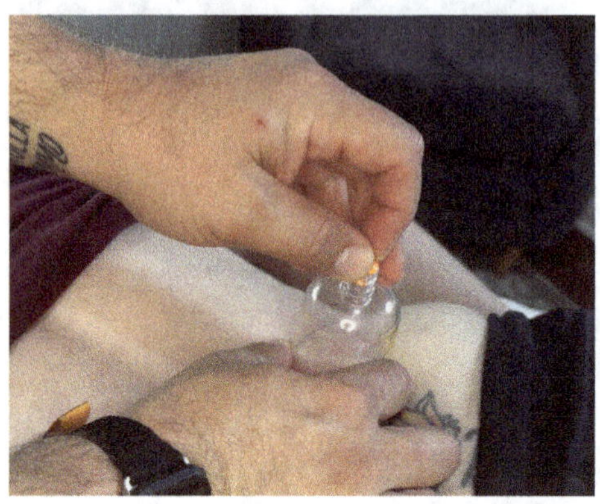

Pump Removal via Releasing the Valve

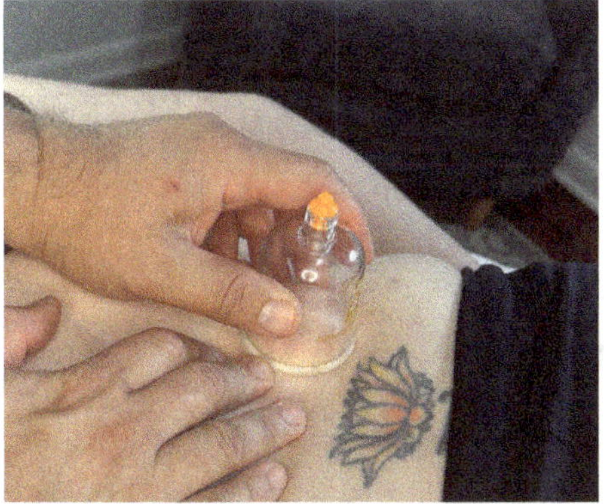

Pump Removal via "Burping"

Do not try to pull any cup straight up off the body. Always release the seal of the cup first.

    b.   Silicone

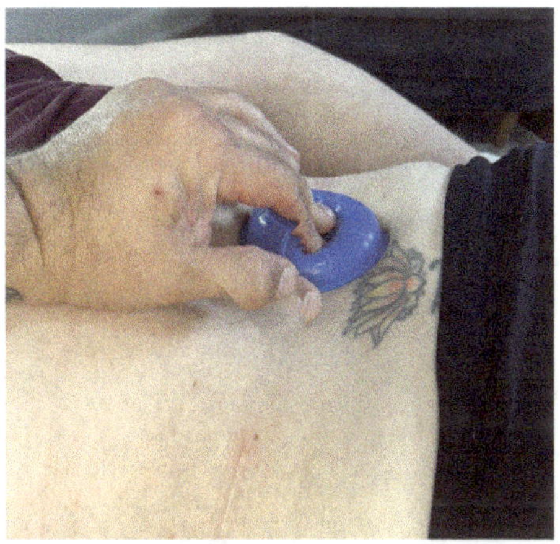

"Burp" to Remove Silicone Cups

To apply these cups, simply place the cup against the body and press the air out. Pressing the cup completely against the skin is going to force the most air out and give the strongest suction. Pressing the cup with less force can allow for a milder treatment.

Removing these cups is simple as well. Just press down on the skin at the outer edge of the cup and slide a finger under the rim. The seal will break. Some people also peel the cup up, but this could be a bit more uncomfortable.

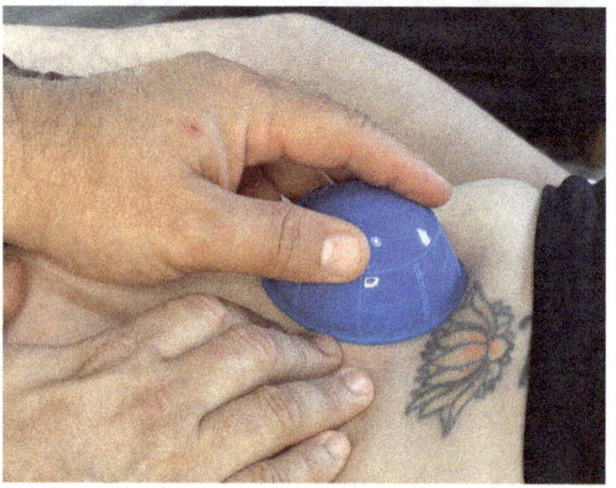

c. Bulb

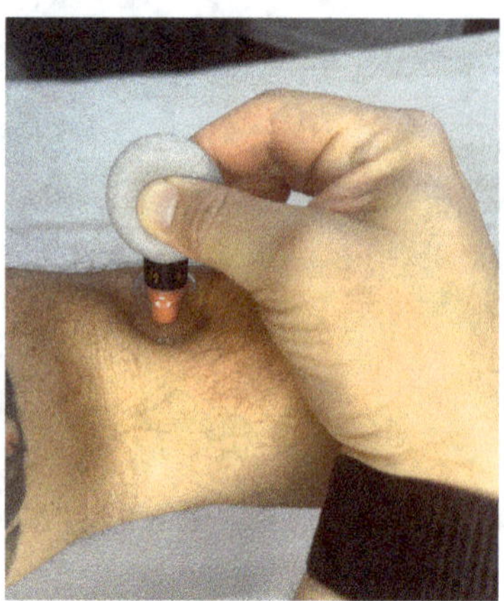

Bulb Style Cup being Applied

To apply this style of cup, simply squeeze the bulb at the top and place it on the skin. Releasing the bulb creates the vacuum that causes the cup to adhere. The stronger the bulb is pressed, the stronger the vacuum effect.

To remove these cups, either slide your finger under the lip of the cup or squeeze the bulb again.

d. Twists

While not difficult to apply, these cups require a little more work to adhere properly. First, make sure the internal screw is all the way down. If the screw is partially up, you may not get enough suction for the cup to stick or the treatment may be too mild.

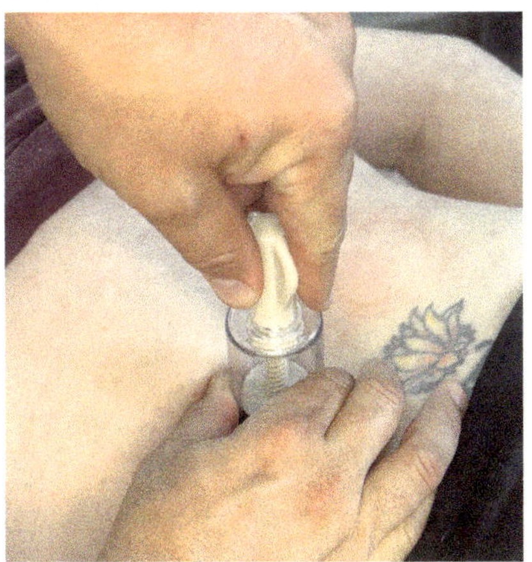

Twist Style Cup being Applied

Place the cup against the skin as you would with every other cup. To get the cup to stick, you need to make sure there is enough downward pressure on the cup while twisting the screw up and away from the body. Sometimes this may require that you use both hands, making these twist-style cups less than ideal for self-treatment. The extra effort, when compared to other styles of cups, may be part of the reason they are less commonly used and harder to find.

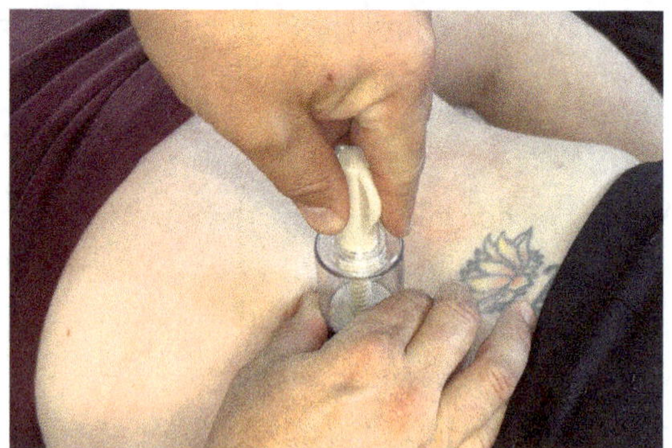

Twist Style Cup can be Removed by Burping or Turning the Other Direction

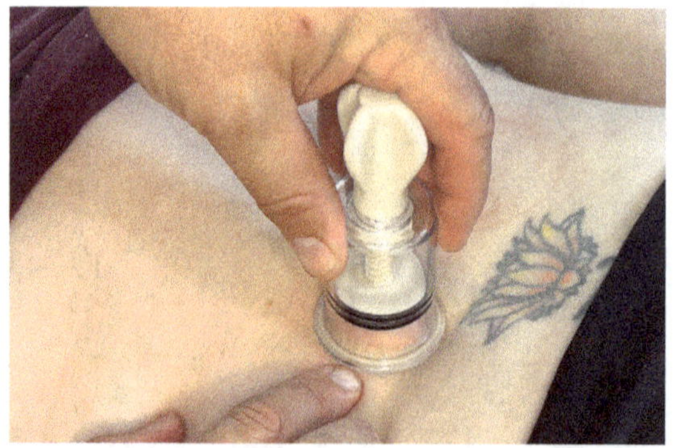

Twist Style Cup Being "Burped"

e. Electronic Combined Therapy

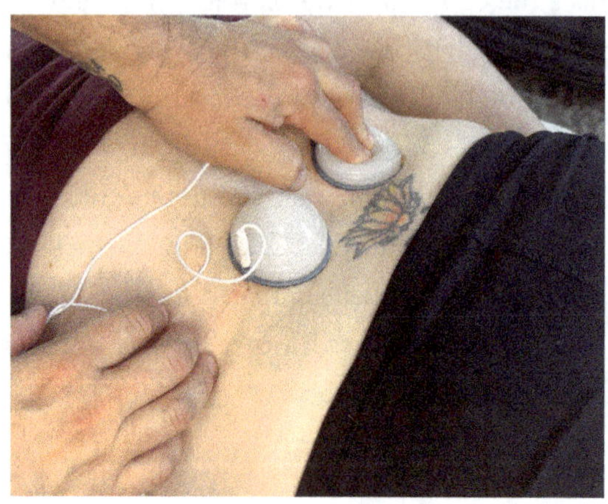

Electric Stimulation Cups Applied

These cups are much newer than the those listed above. However, that does not mean the method for getting them to adhere is different. The cups that combine therapies often have a motorized pump that automatically pumps air out and can be set to a certain intensity level. These newer types of cups usually come with instructions on how to operate them—follow the manufacturer's directions. They should operate with enough similarity to the more common types, and the safety and general guidelines that the instructions lay out should be followed.

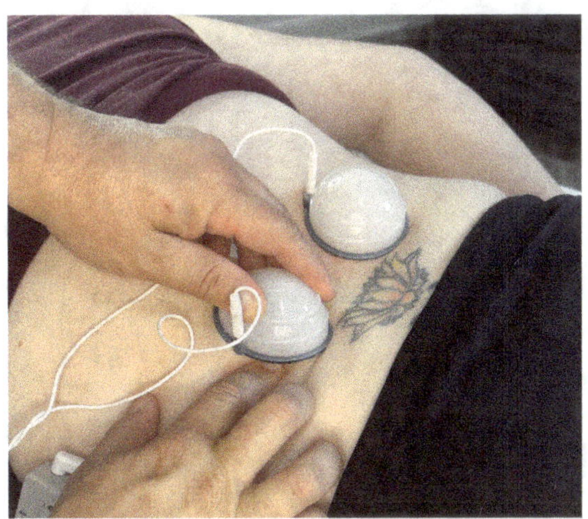

Electric Stimulation Cups Removed

3. *The Treatment*

Once the cups are in place, there isn't much to do. If you are treating yourself, just relax. If you are treating someone else, check in to make sure that they are comfortable. If any cup is uncomfortable, you can remove it and try the area again. If it is still uncomfortable, don't place a cup on that area.

If you are using clear cups, keep an eye on the change of skin color. The "textbook" color would be a deep purplish-red. However, depending on circulation and the health of the blood vessels, some areas might not bruise at all. If you are not using clear cups or can't see a change in the skin, make sure you keep the cups in place for no longer than 15 minutes on any individual spot.

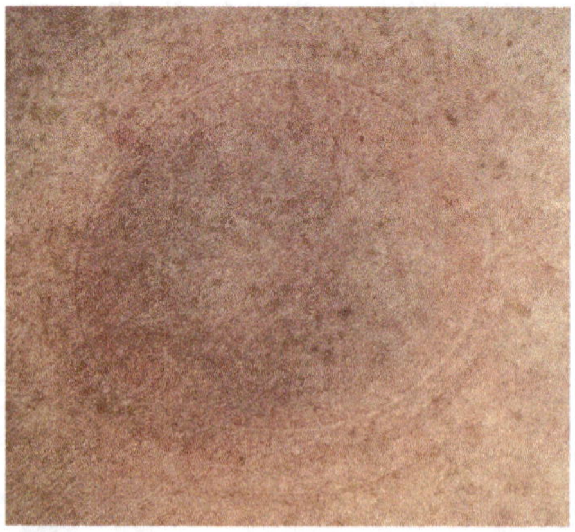

Mild Cupping Marks

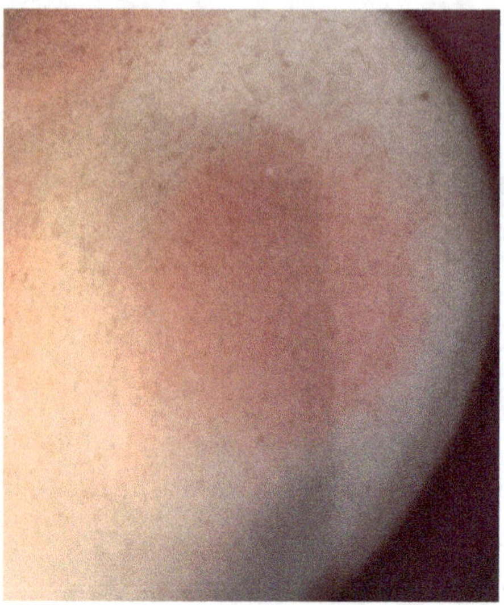

Moderate Cupping Marks

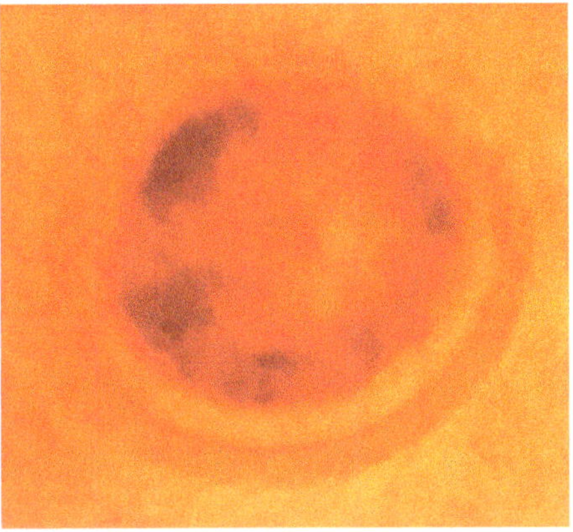

Strong Cupping Marks

When the treatment is done, remove the cups and check the area. Regardless of the amount of bruising in the area, you will notice the skin is depressed where the lip of the cup pressed in and raised in the center, where the mouth of the cup covered the skin. This phenomenon disappears within a few minutes and is a natural response to the pressure from the cup. It is similar to lying on a lounge chair and finding the lines of the chair pressed into your skin when you stand up.

If there is initial bruising, that is to be expected, but it may "set up" over the next few hours and become darker. All of these changes are normal.

SLIDING TECHNIQUE

If you have become proficient at getting cups to stick for static cupping, you are halfway to being proficient at sliding cupping. This method requires the cups to adhere with less pressure than static cupping—if a cup's vacuum is too strong, it will either cause too much pain when you try to slide it or you won't be able to move the cup at all. While this style of cupping can be done on oneself along the legs or maybe an arm, it is usually done on the larger areas like the shoulders and back—more than likely, it will require two people.

This technique is much more intense for the person receiving the treatment than static cupping. It is important to make sure the person being worked on can tolerate it. When the cup moves across the body, the lead edge of the cup depresses the skin. As the area comes under the opening of the cup, it is drawn up—then is forced back down by the other edge of the cup. It feels like a very intense massage.

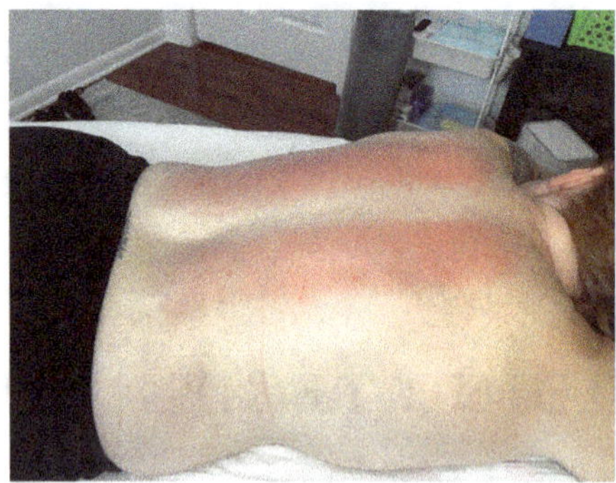

Typical Marks from Sliding Cupping

Sliding cupping usually does not last too long, both because of comfort and how quickly the skin begins to become red. Rather than perfect reddish-purple circles, this leaves long lines of pink-ish red with petechiae, darker dots of red and purple caused by capillaries breaking. This style of cupping is intense; keeping the treatment short and getting constant feedback from the person receiving it can be a very effective way to loosen muscles, release pain, and even open up the chest and lungs.

Here is a step-by-step guide to sliding cupping, that should make it more comfortable.

1.   Apply Oil

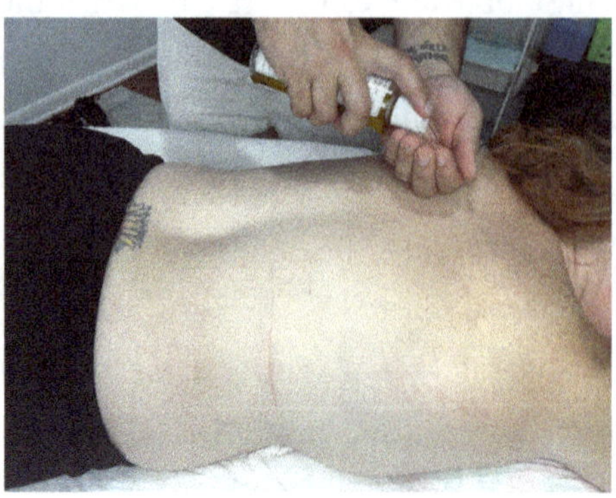

Oil Application

In Chapter 7, we discussed the different types of oils, liniments, and creams that can be applied. For sliding cupping, there must be something on the skin that lubricates, allowing the cup to slide. Make sure there is enough oil applied to the area. It is a good idea to cover a wider area than needed to allow for expanding the treatment without having to stop. The area doesn't need to be dripping but should have more oil than will be absorbed by the skin while working.

2. Apply the Cup

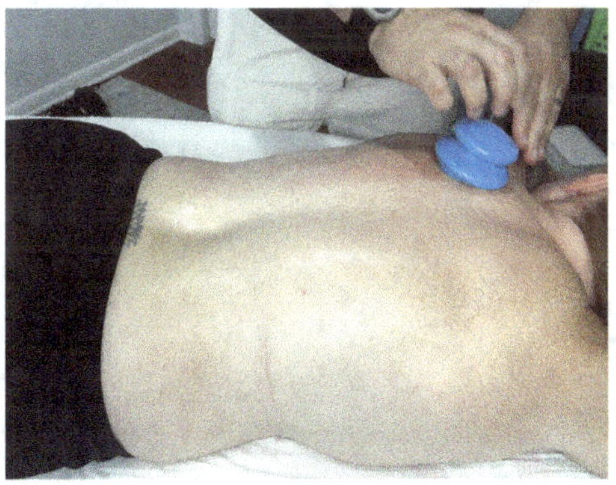

Cup Application

With this technique, most people apply either one cup near the affected area or two cups if the issue is on both sides of the body. If two cups are used—for the hips for instance, you will still only be sliding one cup at a time. Then you switch sides and slide the other cup. The practice of crossing over bones tends to break the suction and feels unpleasant. You do not want multiple cups in one area because there won't be enough room to slide along the surface of the body. Choose one end of a muscle group so you can work up and down the length of the muscle as you move the cup.

When applying a cup for sliding cupping, it is important to get a milder suction so the cup can slide without too much pain. If the suction is too strong, release some of the vacuum, or remove it and try again with less force. Make sure the cup is sturdy enough to slide. As I discussed earlier, soft silicone cups may simply lift off instead of sliding.

3. Sliding

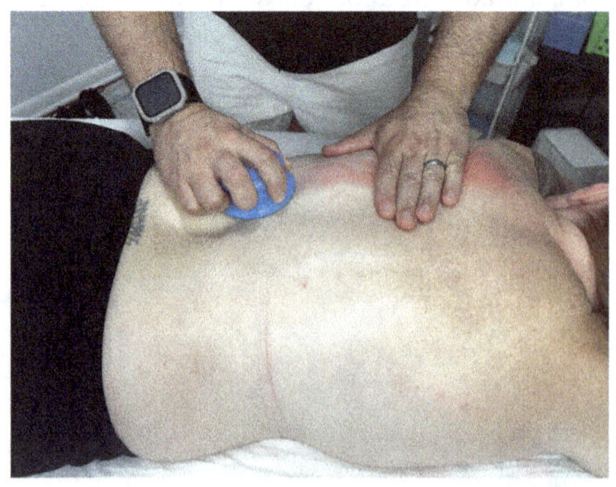

Sliding Cupping with Free Hand Pulling the Skin in the Opposite Direction

Up to this point, the steps of sliding cupping have been almost exactly the same as static cupping. There is oil on the skin and the cup is attached, but these cups need to be applied with less suction.

- Have an idea of the length of the muscle you are working on and in what direction you will be sliding.

- Grasp the cup with the appropriate hand—if you will be sliding to the left, grip the cup with your left hand, etc.

- Use your other hand to apply pressure down and away from the direction you wish to slide the cup. This will stretch the skin and allow the cup to glide easier in the other direction.

- Slide the cup the length of the muscle, making sure that you slide with a smooth motion. If it feels jerky or the person is uncomfortable, the cup may be too tight. If this is the case, try to release some of the pressure or re-apply the cup with less force.

- When you reach the end of the muscle, switch hands and repeat in the opposite direction.

- Repeat these steps back and forth, sliding until there are reddish lines that form along the muscle. There may be varying numbers of red dots, or petechiae, which are good signs.

- Check in frequently with the person receiving the treatment and make sure the pressure is not too intense.

- Sliding may not require many passes, depending on how strong the suction is and how quickly the skin comes up red.

- Remove the cup the same way you would for static cupping.

- If you wish to slide along another muscle, repeat this process on that part of the body.

AREAS TO CUP

Whether you are performing static cupping or sliding cupping, there are some general areas that lend themselves to being cupped. If you are dealing with physical soreness or pain, look not only at the affected area but also at muscle groups and related spots that may be affected. For example, if someone is experiencing soreness along the trapezius muscles, check along the shoulder blade, upper back, and close to the neck. The treatment of any nearby areas with soreness or "knots" will increase the results felt in the main area.

Remember that cupping therapy is more of a "horseshoes and hand grenades" therapy, meaning, it is great to get directly on the problem spot, but if you get close to it, there will still be successful outcomes. This is important when dealing with areas that are too small or rounded for the application of cups. If someone has soreness in the wrist, some smaller cups may fit, but the cups may adhere better further up the forearm where the muscles are bigger and provide a wider surface for attachment. Those muscles attach to the tendons in the wrist. Increasing circulation higher up on the arm will provide a reduction in inflammation in the wrist and fingers.

Before cupping any area, try running your hand over the whole section of the body. Note spots that feel tight or sore and include them in the treatment as well as near or on the affected area. This approach will yield the best results.

In the next section, I will give a brief overview of where you can apply cups, but it is by no means exhaustive. As long as you follow the safety rules and can get the cup to create a vacuum, you can be as creative as you'd like. The photos show some of the more common locations but listen to what the body is telling you about muscle soreness and tight spots.

BACK OF THE BODY

The back side of the body is the most common area for cupping. That is in part because the lower back, neck, and shoulders are often tight and need treatment but it's also because the larger, wide muscles of the back easily lend themselves to cup placement.

There are no hard and fast rules to cupping the back: going by what feels sore and following simple safety rules should give freedom to the practitioner. Just make sure the cups are comfortable when they are placed.

- Lower Back

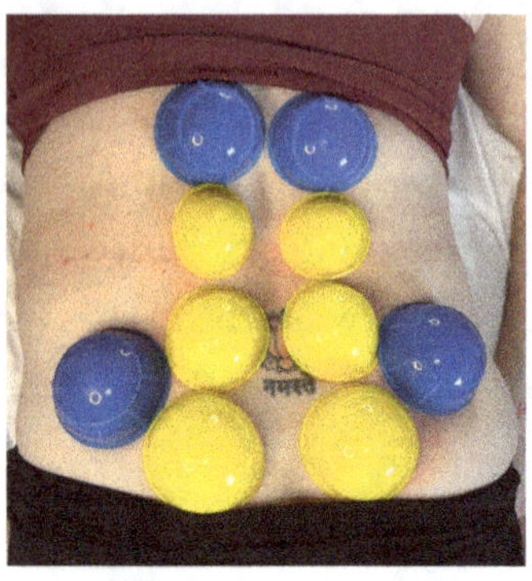

Common Areas to Cup on the Lower Back

Lower back pain might be the reason that most people seek cupping therapy. Not only is it extremely common, but cupping works wonderfully in this area because the large, wide muscles provide plenty of space to attach the cups.

Attach the cups along the spine, on the larger muscles called the erectors that help keep the spine upright. Lower back pain might extend beyond the spine, so cups can also be placed along the hips and upper buttocks and around the sacrum.

• Upper Back

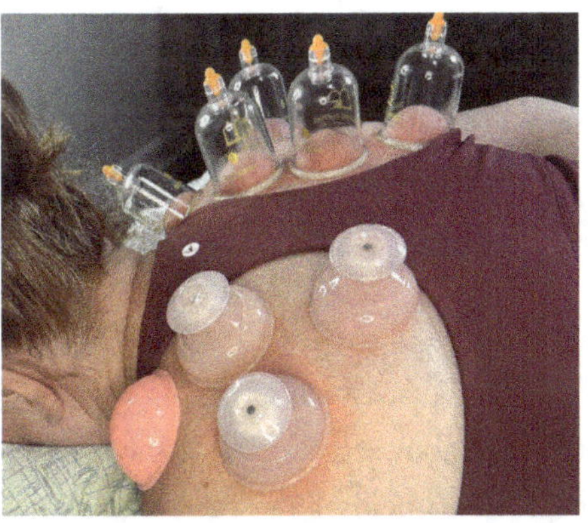

Common Areas to Cup on the Upper Back

This is probably the second most common place for cups. Not only can you treat neck and shoulder pain from the upper back, but the area between the shoulder blades is also right above the lungs and can be cupped for relieving all types of chest congestion and respiratory issues.

While it is difficult to adhere larger cups along the neck, the trapezius muscles at the top of the shoulders are a great place to cup for general stress as well as neck and shoulder pain.

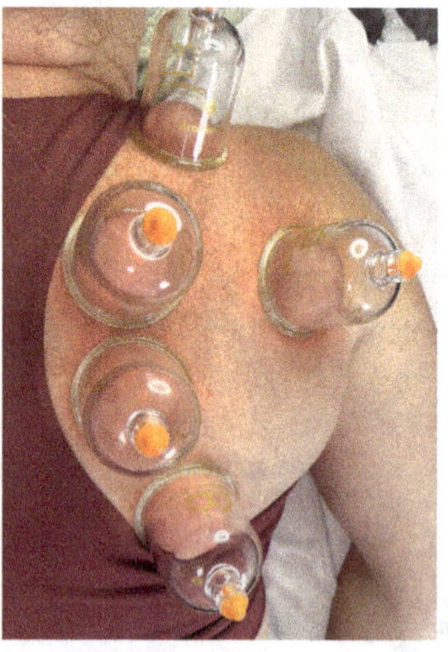

Common Areas to Cup on the Shoulder Blades

For issues that may involve some pain and soreness along the length of the arms, cupping on the shoulder blade and right above the crease of the armpit can really help not only with local tightness but also with circulation in the arms.

• Neck

The neck is a difficult area for attaching cups. The hair along the hairline and the curve of the neck makes it nearly impossible to attach rigid cups; silicone cups are a bit easier to work with. Avoid getting too close to the scalp as the thickness of the hair can prevent a good seal. Using small silicone cups along the spine can help release neck tightness.

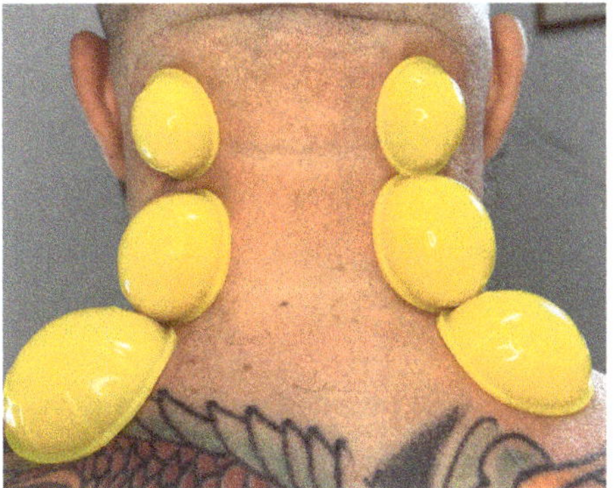

Common Areas to Cup on the Neck

FRONT OF THE BODY

While less common than cupping the back, people have been cupping on the chest for as long as cupping has existed. The pecs, thighs, and the fronts of the shoulders are great areas to cup to help relieve pain and soreness.

Although cupping the abdomen can be helpful for relief from constipation or diarrhea, abdominal cupping has its own rules and should be performed only when appropriate. We will briefly discuss this, but if you are looking for in-depth treatment, please seek a licensed practitioner.

- Chest

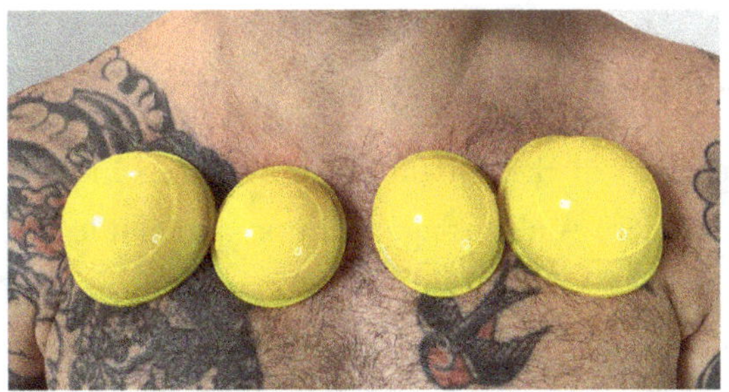

Common Areas to Cup on the Chest

Areas including the front of the shoulders, the upper chest, and the front edge of the trapezius muscles can be cupped to relieve chest congestion or pain in the chest muscles. **Note:** If you are working on a female, be sure to avoid breast tissue. Keep the cups closer to the collarbones and make sure that the cups stay on muscle tissue.

If you are using cups for chest congestion, you can cup both the upper chest and the upper back, and there are two ways to do it. Have the person sit up straight if you want to treat the chest and back at the same time. Have the person lie down to treat the front and back separately in stages.

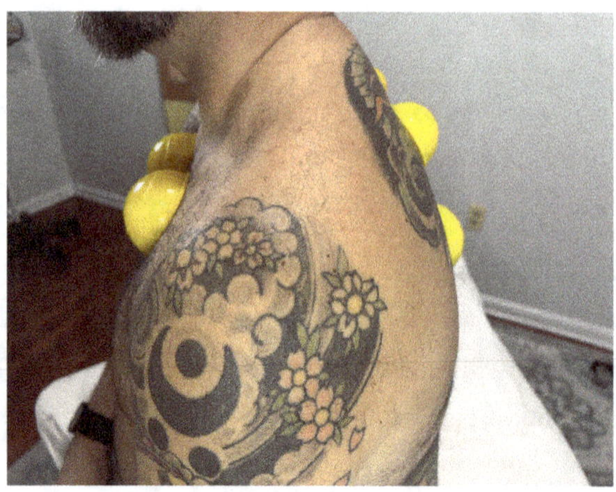

Cupping on the Chest and Back while Sitting

THE LIMBS

Many people experience tightness and soreness in their arms and legs. If the cups you're using can fit on arm and leg muscles and hold a good seal, it's worth trying to attach them to bring more circulation to the sore areas. However, if the curve of the area is too tight, there is excessive body hair that even using oil will not help, or the cup keeps falling off, it may be easier to cup points on the trunk of the body that will open circulation to these areas.

Having a wide variety of cup sizes available will allow you to reach more areas for treatment. Simple safety precautions should still be followed, but it is generally safe to cup on the limbs.

- Thighs

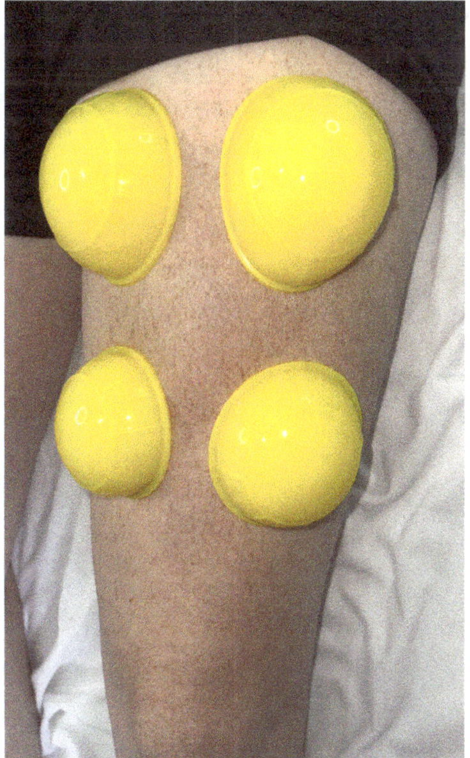

Cupping the on the Quads

If you are a runner, a weightlifter, or you're on your feet at work, your thighs can get very tight. All surfaces of the thigh can receive cupping. It is great for the quads, hamstrings, and IT (iliotibial) bands that run along the outside of the leg. These bulky muscles have everything required of a good surface for cupping; they are long, generally flat, and wide. You may require some oil or lotion if the areas are hairy.

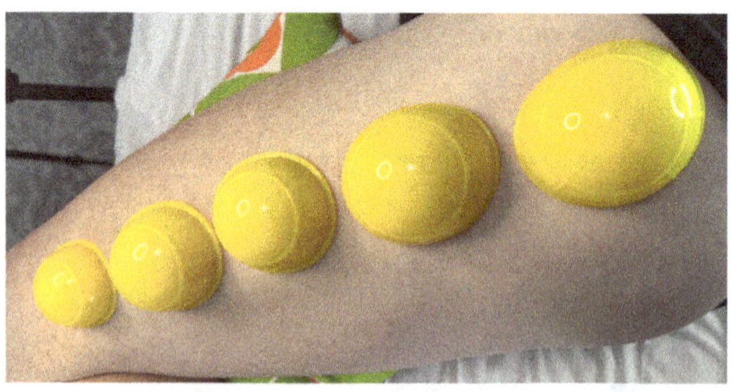

Cupping on the IT Band

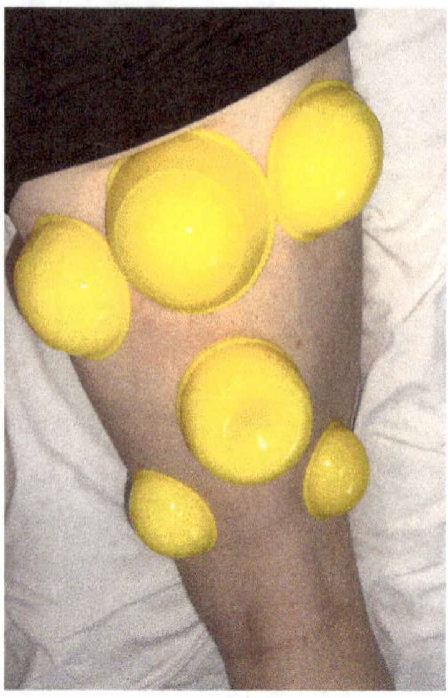

Typical Cupping on the Hamstrings

There are some specific guidelines for the thighs, all of which concern the level of pain that strong cupping or sliding cupping can cause in this area:

- Do not cup around the back of the knee where there is a superficial popliteal artery. You do not want to damage that.

- Sliding cupping must be done with caution along the legs as the area can be surprisingly sensitive.

- Go lightly if you want to work on the adductors—muscles on the inside of the thigh—and don't get too close to the groin. You do not want to accidentally bump into the genitals or catch them with the cups.

- Calves

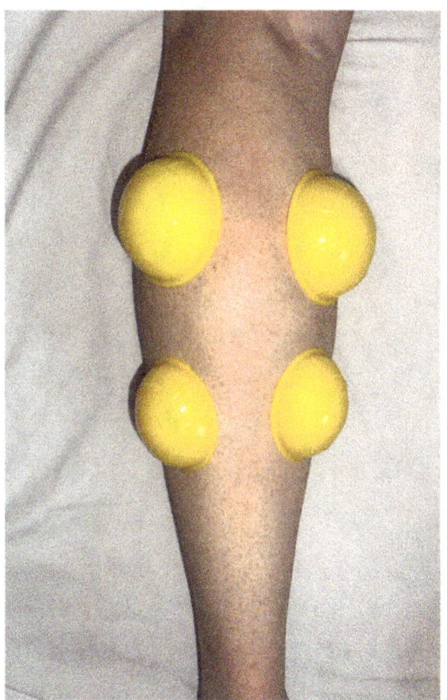

Typical Cupping on the Calves

When cupping the calves, it is a good idea to stay on the posterior of the lower leg. Look for spots along the wider gastrocnemius muscle, which is composed of two bulky heads on the inside and outside of the calf. You need to choose small enough cups to fit, and some kind of oil will help the cups stick. Avoid the shin and the Achilles tendon. Cupping has a better effect on muscles than on tendons.

- Feet

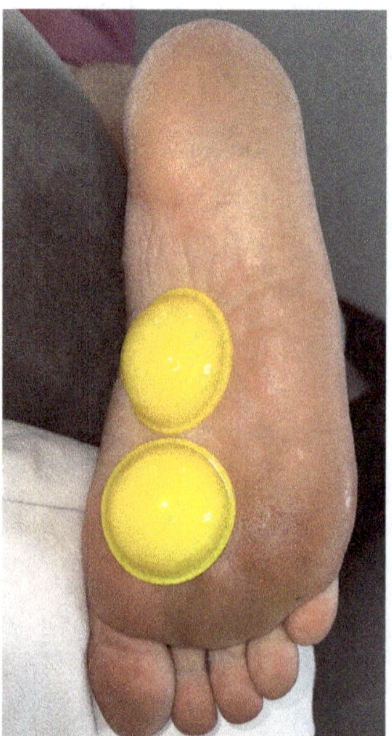

Cups on Feet

There is no question that aching feet are a common complaint, but many professionals, myself included, prefer to avoid cupping the soles of the feet. The problem is the difficulty in getting cups, even small ones, to adhere to the feet. Adding additional oil may be helpful and closer to the ball of the foot tends to work better than the harder, thicker heel. Even with strong initial suction these cups will frequently loosen on their own. There's no harm in trying it if you want to, but you might quickly decide to forgo the frustration and get yourself a good foot massage instead.

- Forearms

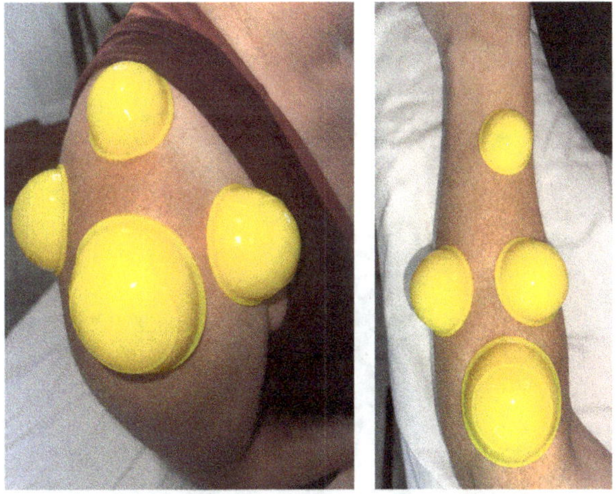

Typical Cupping on the Forearms and Upper Arms

The forearms can be cupped following a similar logic to cupping the calves. You are more likely to get cups to attach to the muscles closer to the elbow, which are bigger than the muscles near the wrist. Small cups can be placed closer to the wrist, but attaching cups to the belly of the bigger muscles will also provide significant reduction in pain and soreness in the wrist area.

NON-PAIN ISSUES

Cupping may be helpful for a wider variety of conditions than just pain and soreness. However, when we move internally or discuss stress, we we're talking about deeper organs or how to trigger a calming response in the mind through various areas of the body. While cupping can sometimes help, as with the muscular symptoms, if you do not see continued improvement, please seek a licensed healthcare practitioner.

- Stress

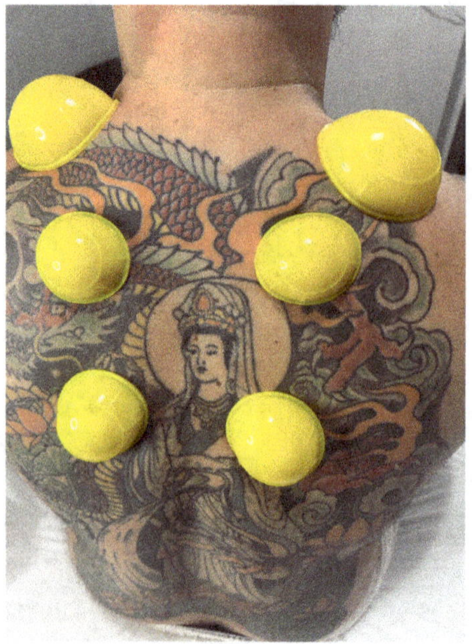

Areas to Cup to Relieve Stress

Stress is one of the big reasons that people seek cupping. Stress does not have a centralized location, but people do feel it in their bodies. For many, this may be the neck and shoulders, between the shoulder blades, and the lower back. All of these sites are perfect for cupping. Place the cups as you would for any pain condition. Sometimes it may be helpful to cup along both sides of the spine from the top of the shoulders down to the hips.

- Digestion

Cupping on the abdomen is done less widely, but it can help a variety of digestive issues. Static cupping brings more blood flow to the intestines, promoting proper peristalsis (movement of the muscles in the tract) and reduction of abdominal pain. Apply the cups to any tender areas that you find by pressing on the belly. The treatment time on the abdomen is usually much shorter than in other areas. A few minutes should be enough, and the usual red marks may not appear.

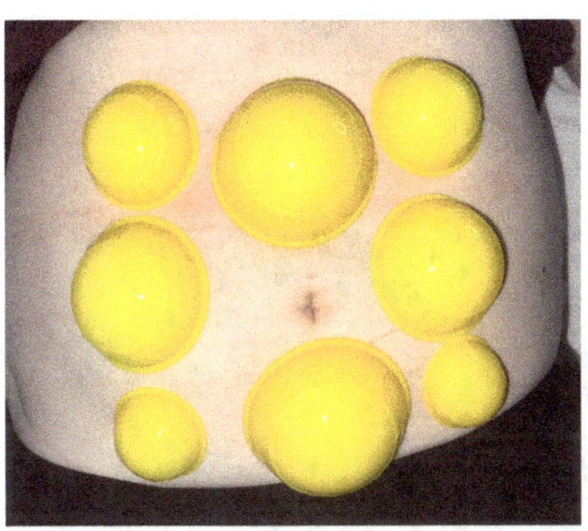

Common Areas to Cup for Digestion

People have used sliding cupping to help with constipation by following the path of the large intestine.

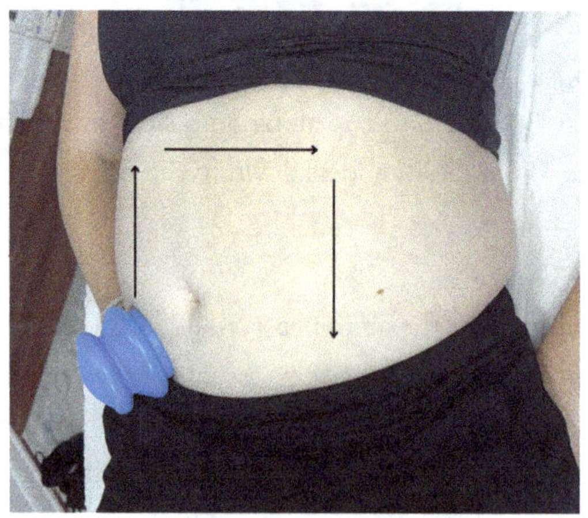

Sliding for Constipation (clockwise)

To do this, start at the lower right side of the abdomen. Slide the cup upward toward the rib cage, then slide to the left side of the abdomen following the lower edge of the ribs. Finally, slide downward on the left side of the abdomen. Remember to have a supporting hand pulling the skin in the opposite direction of the cup. Repeat this a few times.

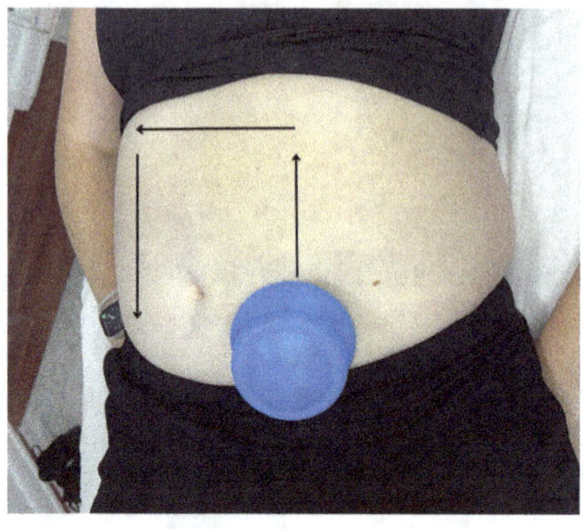

Sliding for Diarrhea (counterclockwise)

If someone is suffering from diarrhea, do the exact opposite on the pathway of the large intestine. Starting at the lower left side of the abdomen, slide upward toward the rib cage, then to the right along the lower edge of the ribs, then down the right side.

- Sinus Congestion

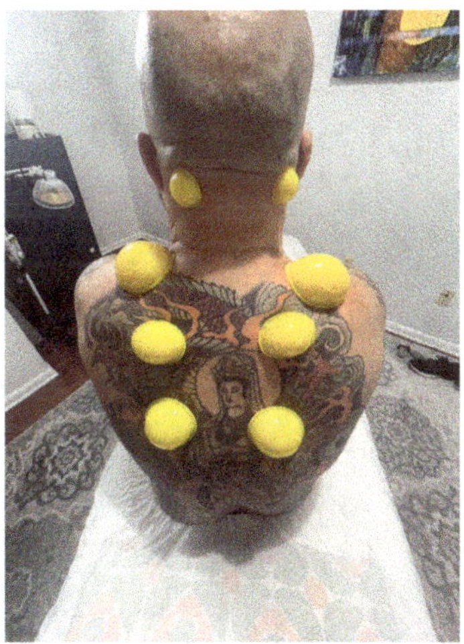

Cupping on Neck and Upper Back for Sinus Issues

Cupping specific areas of the upper chest can help with some sinus issues. If you have small enough cups, you can also work the top of the trapezius muscles and the posterior muscles of the neck up to the hairline—as close as you can get without the hair interfering. This is another area where you will cup for a shorter amount of time. Sliding can be performed, but the cups are likely to fall off. If you slide, put more emphasis on the downward motion—from the hairline toward the shoulders.

WHAT DO THE BRUISES "MEAN"?

EXPLAINING A CUPPING MARK CHART

For as long as I have been performing cupping, people have asked me questions about the marks. These questions often revolve around the darkness of the color. Some examples include:

- "Does it mean something if the marks are dark?"

- "How come I don't bruise on my lower back, but my shoulders turn purple?"

- "How come most marks go away in a day but this one area sticks around for longer than a week?"

- "Why did my friends' bruises get super dark, but mine barely turned red?"

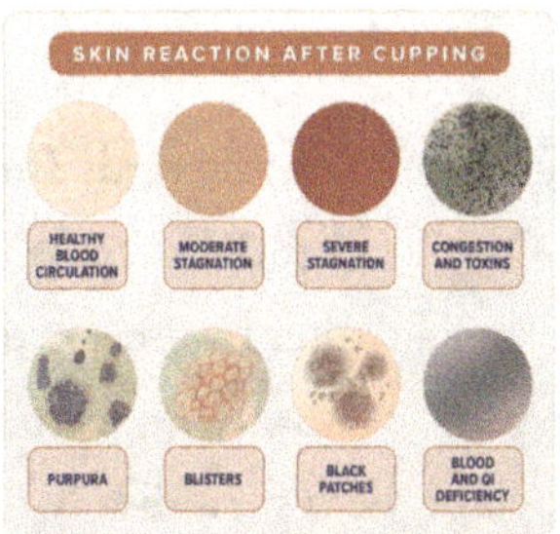

A typical chart showing the possible meanings of cupping marks

These are all valid questions. If you've seen any Instagram, Facebook, or Pinterest charts that many of my colleagues share, you might have read that the darker the bruise the more "blood stagnation" is prevalent. Some even claim that if you don't bruise in an area, you are "blood deficient." These statements are confusing because they don't tell the whole story—those charts are meant to quickly educate someone on the *possible* reasons why your body responds in a certain fashion.

In East Asian medicine, you cannot hang a complete diagnosis on one single sign or symptom, which is what a simple chart does. Is it wrong? Not exactly, but there are many reasons why one cupping mark may be darker than another nearby.

Before we get into what the various colors can roughly "mean," we should take a look at some of the factors that will influence how dark those bruises get.

- Strength of Suction

    The amount of suction an individual cup has will greatly alter the color of a mark. Stronger suction will often create darker marks. Once you are comfortable with whatever cupping set you use, you should get a feel for the strength of its suction and how you can keep the suction consistent to better control outcomes.

- Duration of Treatment

    This one is pretty straightforward: The longer the cups are in place, the more potential there is for the capillaries to rupture, causing a darker bruise. If you have opaque cups and cannot see the skin, it might be a good idea to remove and replace them periodically during the treatment to make sure you don't overdo it.

- Vascular Health

  One person's capillaries may be stronger- or weaker-walled than another's, depending on their age and health. In addition, the overall strength of the smaller blood vessels will play into how dark the circles may appear.

- Vascular Density

  Certain areas of the body have a higher volume of blood vessels than others. For instance, the areas just below the crest of the hips not only have more fat but also have less blood-vessel density and tend to bruise less. Areas such as the back of the shoulder blade usually become quite dark due to how many blood vessels innervate that tissue.

- Fat

  You should have fat on your body, and certain areas should have more of it. These areas may have fewer superficial blood vessels and may not get as dark when cupped.

- Type of Cup Used

  Different types of cups may provide a stronger treatment. While stronger doesn't necessarily mean better, it often does mean darker cupping marks. All cupping sessions should be tolerable. Do not make them a "no pain, no gain" situation.

- The Timing of When the Cups Are Placed

  Watching the Olympics might make you have cup-mark

envy. The athletes have perfect reddish-purple circles everywhere. One big reason for this may be that they are getting treated shortly after working out. The blood is coursing through their bodies and more of it is at the surface, adding to the darkness of their cupping marks.

- Whether or Not the Person Exercises

People who exercise more not only develop more muscle, but they also develop more blood vessels to carry blood to and from the muscles. This doesn't only apply to people who lift weights to build muscle mass, it also applies to people who do endurance events where the muscles may not be bulky but are very toned.

- Previous Injury in the Area

In traditional Chinese medicine, injuries and circulation issues often lead to a concept called "blood stagnation." If we look at this through a modern lens, we can see that when there is poor circulation in an area, blood does not travel in and out efficiently, so the tissue not only lacks nutrients and fresh oxygen but also has metabolic waste and inflammatory compounds building up in it. Areas around damaged tissue can have quite a bit of blood stasis and can yield very dark circles.

Now that we see that there are many factors that can affect how "bruised" the treatment can leave a person, we will discuss what those different colors *may* mean.

- Red to Dark Red/Purple Marks

It seems as though anyone requesting cupping *wants* very

dark marks to show that the cupping had an effect. While most often there will be some darkening at the cupping site, the color of the cupping mark does not necessarily correlate to how successful the session will be in providing relief.

The easy and often overutilized comment about dark red or purple marks is that they mean there is stagnation in the area. Stagnation in this sense comes from traditional Chinese medicine and refers to the fact that blood is not smoothly flowing through the area.

We usually see the darkest spots near areas that have a good amount of vasculature near the surface, near an injured or affected area, or where there is muscle tightness. Many of these situations do lend themselves to a diagnosis of blood stagnation, but as we discussed previously, there are many variables.

Dark marks are often a good indication that cupping was appropriate in that area and the marks are a "textbook" reaction. Another commonly used phrase that we hear when there is a good amount of redness at the cupping site is that the area "needed it." Though not wrong, that statement only pinpoints one reason for marks becoming dark red.

- No Bruising

Some people are disappointed if there are no marks even after an intense cupping session. Remember, bruising is not an indication of results. Results may be great without the marks.

As we've discussed, in traditional Chinese medicine, blood stasis can be the reason that dark circles appear. Similarly, TCM suggests blood deficiency as a reason that no marks appear. Blood deficiency is a concept that implies the lack of good quality blood either locally or throughout the whole body. Signs would include some generalized weakness: a pale tongue for instance, or, in women, scant periods. Once again, this is only one possible reason that there may be little to no color where a cup was placed.

Many other reasons exist as well, the most common being a lack of vasculature in the area, low suction in the cups, or removal of cups before they had time to cause a bruise. Whatever the reason, look more for relief of the symptoms and let that be the guide for judging the effectiveness of the treatment.

• Blisters

Blisters should be an extremely rare occurrence in cupping. In my 22 years of clinical practice, performing cupping on patients multiple times a day, I have had only two cases in which I saw blisters form. If you follow the general practice guidelines about the strength and duration of a cupping session, you should be able to avoid ever having to deal with blisters. They usually occur if the cups have been on too long or the suction was too strong.

In some cases, blisters may be associated with the Chinese medical term "dampness," which is a condition that is heavy, slow-moving, and wet. Usually, symptoms here can include excess body weight, edema, and lethargy. These symptoms normally appear after a long-standing imbalance, such as improper digestion from eating fried foods or dairy.

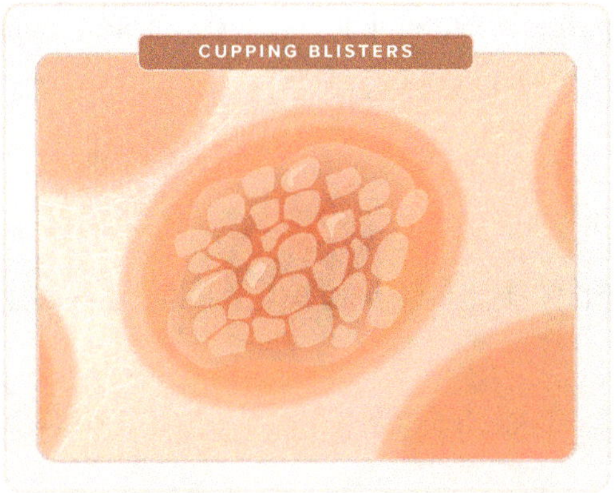

Although very rare, cupping may cause blisters

Classically, the symptoms may worsen if someone is living in a damp environment—such as a basement apartment—or frequently has to work in the rain. While the concept of dampness is used to point to a collection of symptoms that may or may not be present, it does not mean cupping is forbidden. It does mean proceeding with caution when doing so. That being said, of the two cases of blistering that I've experienced, one was in a relatively healthy patient with no signs of dampness.

Although blistering is an extremely rare issue, it is important to mention how to take care of blisters if they do occur.

If blisters form and you notice them through clear cups, remove *all the cups* immediately. Usually, blistering won't occur under every cup, but it is better to be safe than sorry. Blisters will usually look like they are filled with a clear or straw-colored fluid. In even rarer cases, blood blisters can form that will be the same size but filled with blood. In either situation, blisters are very delicate and can easily pop. Avoid popping them.

Here is a step-by-step approach to dealing with blisters from cupping:

1. Clean the area with water and soap but be very gentle.

2. Dry the area with clean gauze.

3. Cover the area with a large bandage or sterile gauze and medical tape.

4. Keep the area clean and dry so that the blisters will pop on their own.

The area will take longer to heal than normal bruising. Avoid cupping therapy during that time. Once the blisters pop, keep the dressings clean and apply antibiotic cream to the area. If anything looks infected or unhealthy, seek medical care.

This section is not meant to scare people away from cupping, merely to make practitioners aware that blistering may occur, no matter how rare the occurrence. If it happens, check your technique and make sure you are not putting the cups on too strongly or leaving them for too long. Most silicone cups are not able to create that strong a vacuum, but still, keep the cups in one area for under 15 minutes.

AFTER THE TREATMENT

Sometimes, cupping gives people near-instantaneous relief. Whether because of a reduction in pain or just relaxation, people can usually feel some change by the time they are up and moving around. Other times, people notice an effect either a few hours later or the next day. Any forward progress is good, and it is important to remember that this is a therapy, not a "magic bullet" offering an immediate cure. Results to expect from a session are not written in stone and can vary widely from treatment to treatment.

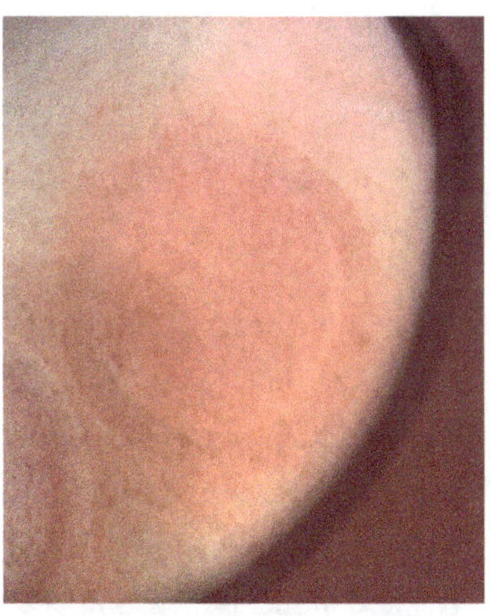

Ridge from Cupping Immediately After Removal

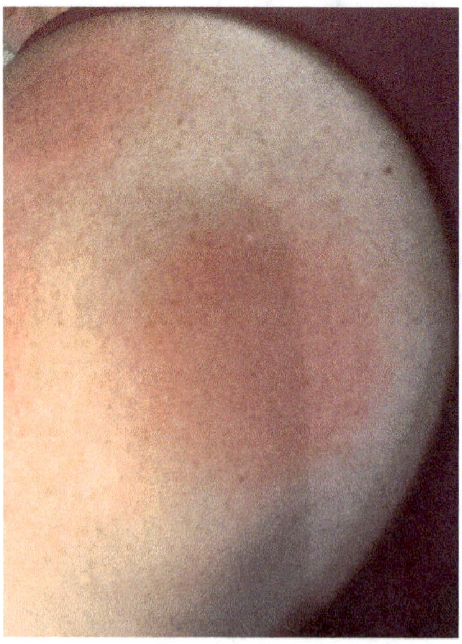

No Ridge after a Few Minutes

When the cups first come off, there is normally a "bruised" raised area where the opening of the cup was and a depressed ring where the lip of the cup pressed into the skin. I often tell people this is like lying on a folding beach chair and then, when you get up, finding lines on your skin. The compression of the lip and the suction from the cup moves underlying fluids in the body. Once the cup is removed, the unevenness of the skin takes a couple of minutes to return to normal.

Some people recommend increasing water intake after a cupping session because moving the skin, fascia, and muscles move metabolic waste and inflammation out of the tissue. Increasing the amount of water you drink after any manual therapy, such as cupping or massage, helps flush those compounds to the core to be processed by the liver and kidneys. Increasing water consumption allows more fluid in the body to flush out what many therapists will refer to as "toxins." I tend to avoid that word as it's something anyone and everyone says regarding health trends, while failing to back up that claim. There is no evidence for "flushing out toxins," but one glass of water will not hurt.

Once done, the color of the areas that were cupped can range in intensity. As we discussed previously, there is no need to worry about the particular shade of the marks. However, cupping marks are usually at their darkest a couple of hours after the session when enough blood has circulated to the area. Some of these marks may be gone within a day or two while other darker marks may last more than a week. If you plan on regular cupping sessions, it's best to leave areas that have not yet resolved from the previous session alone. You can choose areas nearby to continue working on the same muscle groups without over-treating.

Sometimes, though rarely, the worked areas may feel sore, as if they received an intense massage. This soreness may last several hours, and if it is too intense a warm shower and some stretching may alleviate it. The soreness can be due to increased blood flow out of the area or moving metabolic waste and inflammation. It is generally a good sign.

When the session is over, listen to your body but—usually—you won't need to alter your schedule afterward. Resume the activities of daily life, but keep in mind that even if an injured area feels better after a session, it needs to continue to heal and that takes time, so be gentle with it. For example, if your lower back was in pain and cupping alleviated it and you feel good enough to go to the gym, you can do so. However, be careful with any exercise that may affect the lower back. In other words, do not try to set a personal record for a deadlift.

Other than these few considerations, post-treatment care is minimal. Some people like to check on the marks daily to track how soon they can re-treat an area, but that doesn't take more than a few seconds.

CLEANING YOUR CUPS

Keeping your cups clean may seem like an afterthought. If you are the only one using them, why should it matter? Even though there is less cleaning involved if you are only using them on yourself, dead skin, oils, and any bacteria that sits on your body end up sitting in those cups. If you are treating your back with cupping, you are going to need help getting the cups on your back, which means that you may be sharing the kit with family and friends. Cleaning the cups keeps you and anyone using them healthy and safe.

- Professional Cleaning

  In a clinical situation, there are specific protocols to make sure the cups are not only free from oils and dead skin, but also sterilized completely so germs are not passed from one patient to another. Often, clinics also perform acupuncture or wet cupping, and blood may come in contact with the cups.

  Any cleaning protocol must be able to kill any blood-borne pathogens along with making the cups shiny and clean. This is usually a multistep process designed to remove the initial debris from the cups, a sterilizing agent, and then another wash. While glass cups used during fire cupping hold up well to this, the plastics used in pump-style cupping kits tend not to do well with a hospital-strength agent. They quickly become discolored and—though clean—they appear opaque and start to break down. Other materials such as silicone may hold up to the cleaning, but in general, a home kit requires a less-intense cleaning protocol.

- Keeping Your Cups Clean at Home

While they do not need to be sterilized, they should be cleaned thoroughly between uses. Even if they are used solely by one person, skin and body oil can build up over time, making the cups visibly dirty. If you are using oils and liniments, there is a possibility that some of them could degrade plastic cups if not cleaned properly as well.

Over the years, I have seen and heard several opinions on cleaning cups at home. Some sound more thorough than others. In most cases, whatever you choose to do, you should, at the bare minimum, wash them with dish soap and water to remove oils and skin cells as well as keeping them clean to look at. If you are the only one using the cups, washing with dish soap and water may be enough to keep the cups clean and safe. If you are using a set of cups that has a hand pump, the pump will not need to be cleaned, but you do want to be certain that the valve on the cups dries thoroughly to ensure that it stays intact.

Some people use the dishwasher to clean cups. This approach should remove the oil and skin cells but could possibly destroy some plastic cups if you use a high-temperature setting. This will only happen with lower quality cups, but it is worth testing with one plastic cup first before throwing your whole kit in the dishwasher. Try placing plastic cups on the upper rack, as it is cooler than the bottom. You may wish to give the cups an initial handwashing as well, to get rid of any debris that you don't want to come in contact with your dishes.

Disinfecting wipes provide a great additional layer of cleaning to ensure you take care of most of the germs. Any brand of wipe that claims to kill a large percentage of bacteria should do the job well. Some may do a better job than others with removing oils, so handwashing may be necessary either before or after using the wipes. If you are using plastic cups or cups that have rubber on them, you may want to rinse these after the wipes to avoid breakdown of the material.

Bleach seems to be a good overall cleaner if you have the time to allow the cups to soak after use. Years ago, a 10 percent bleach solution was recommended as the preferred sterilizing agent for clinically used cups. This can be used at home too. It is a multiple-step process that includes a quick handwash to remove oil, followed by a 20-minute soak in the 10 percent bleach solution, and then finishing with a rinse to wash off any bleach. If you plan on using the cups on people outside of your family or are really concerned about germs, this is the best option for cleaning cups. With bleach, you may slowly wear down some plastic or rubber on cups, so remember to inspect them frequently.

CLOSING COMMENTS

This book is meant to help keep alive a traditional therapy that was often performed at home. Hopefully, you found it educational without it sounding like a textbook. It was my intention to discuss the styles of cups that do not need to be used with fire to open up this healing practice to more people who may have been put off by the thought of burning their homes down.

I want to thank you for reading this book and I sincerely hope you take action and try the techniques discussed in these pages. While I am a clinician and want my practice to stay busy, the better people take care of themselves and their loved ones, the better their lives will be, which will make the work of every healthcare professional's job much easier.

When we feel good, we are better people. At the risk of sounding too "out there," this will resonate and help the health of humanity as a whole.

One of the goals in writing this was to democratize, decentralize, and demonetize one aspect of healthcare. These are three of Peter Diamandis and Stephen Koltar's six Ds of Technological Disruption. While a 4,000-year-old technique has little to do with modern technology, the principles still hold true.

Democratizing it by allowing everyone to participate in this practice.

Decentralizing it by allowing anyone, anywhere to perform this technique without the need to find a clinic or center that performs it.

Demonetizing it in that after buying some basic supplies there is no need to spend money on practitioners. A decent cupping set will last a long time.

Please practice and share this technique with others, and when you do, remember that you are now part of the history of one of the oldest therapies on the planet!

BIBLIOGRAPHY

1. Al-Bedah, A., Elsubai, I. S., Qureshi, N. A., Aboushanab, T. S., Ali, G., El-Olemy, A. T., Khalil, A., Khalil, M., and Alqaed, M. S. (2018). The medical perspective of cupping therapy: Effects and mechanisms of action. Journal of traditional and complementary medicine, 9(2), 90–97. https://doi.org/10.1016/j.jtcme.2018.03.003

2. Rochat De La Vallee, Elisabeth. *Pregnancy and Gestation in Chinese Classical Text*, Monkey Press, 2007

3. Lim D. W., Kim J. G., Han T., Jung S. K., Lim E. Y., Han D., Kim Y. T. Analgesic Effect of Ilex paraguariensis Extract on Postoperative and Neuropathic Pain in Rats. Biol Pharm Bull. 2015;38(10):1573-9. doi: 10.1248/bpb.b15-00360. Epub 2015 Jul 31. PMID: 26228736.

RESOURCES

For more information on cupping please go to:
thecuppingbook.com

For more information about my clinic, classes, seminars and events please go to:
charmcityintegrative.com

For more information about my clinic, please go to:
charmcityintegrative.com

Connect with me on social media:

Facebook:
www.facebook.com/CharmCityIntegrative

Twitter:
twitter.com/CCIntegrative

Instagram:
www.instagram.com/ccintegrative

YouTube:
www.youtube.com/c/CharmCityIntegrativeHealthBaltimore

Medium:
medium.com/@charmcityintegrative

ABOUT THE AUTHOR

Dr. Tom Ingegno, DACM has more than 22 years of experience in the integrative and functional medicine space. He owns and operates Charm City Integrative Health, a multifaceted clinic that NYT bestseller and futurist David Houle called, the "Future of Medicine," in Baltimore Maryland. This clinic provides a multidimensional approach to reducing inflammation, improving circulation, and regulating the immune system. Tom has taught at two prestigious schools for East Asian medicine, is a published author, and has helped expand the scope for the practice of acupuncture with his role as chairman of the Maryland State Board of Acupuncture. He served as director of a chain of wellness centers in the mid-Atlantic, developing treatment protocols and managing practitioners. Dr. Tom has been featured in both consumer and professional media, spreading his message of health using modern research, traditional practices, and humor to make complex theories and treatments understandable. His professional passion is to help patients and like-minded practitioners develop no-nonsense practices to allow people to thrive.

ACKNOWLEDGMENTS

I would like to thank all the people that helped in the creation of this text.

Thank you to my office staff for being supportive and creating the time and space for me to be able to step out of the clinic to finish this book, even though it took much longer than anticipated.

Thank you to the brilliant calligrapher Eri Takase from stockkanji.com for the beautiful phrase that is both the epigraph to this book and a custom scroll that is a focal point in our office.

Thank you to the amazing team at BookLaunchers.com who have helped me finally cross the finish line and make this idea a reality.